PLAY HARD EAT RIGHT

A Parents' Guide
to Sports Nutrition
for Children

The American Dietetic Association is the largest group of food and nutrition professionals in the world. As the advocate of the profession, the ADA serves the public by promoting optimal nutrition, health, and well-being. For expert answers to your nutrition quesions, call the ADA/National Center for Nutrition and Dietetics Hot Line at (800) 366-1655, and speak directly with a registered dietitian (RD), listen to recorded messages, or obtain a referral to an RD in your area.

JOHN WILEY & SONS, INC.

New York / Chichester / Weinheim / Brisbane / Singapore / Toronto

Play Hard, Eat Right. ©1995, The American Dietetic Association.

Library of Congress Cataloging-in-Publication Data

Jennings, Debbi Sowell.
Play hard, eat right: a parents' guide to sports nutrition for children/ Debbi Sowell Jennings, Suzanne Nelson Steen.

p.   cm.

ISBN 0-471-34695-0
1. Children—Nutrition. 2. Athletes—Nutrition.
I. Steen, Suzanne Nelson. II. Title.

RJ206.J46   1995
613.2'082—dc20   95-16308
                                                  CIP

Edited by: Jeff Braun
Cover Design: MacLean and Tuminelly
Cover Photograph: Paul Lundquist
Production Artist: Janet Hogge
Art/Production Manager: Claire Lewis

Debbi Sowell Jennings, MS, RD
*Pediatric Nutrition Practice Group of
The American Dietetic Association
Department of Pediatrics, University of Alabama at
Birmingham, Birmingham, Alabama*

Suzanne Nelson Steen, DSc, RD
*Sports, Cardiovascular, and Wellness Nutritionist Practice
Group of The American Dietetic Association
University of Pennsylvania School of Medicine
Department of Psychiatry
Philadelphia, Pennsylvania*

The American Dietetic Association

Contributors
Jacqueline R. Berning, MS, RD, Ginny B. Kisler, MS, RD,
Barbara H. Lummis, MS, RD, Josephine Connolly-Schoonen,
MS, RD, Maria H. Seman, MS, RD, Laura B. Szekely, MS, RD,
DeAnn Whitmire, MS, RD

Reviewers
M. T. DiFerante, MPH, RD, Alice Lindeman, PhD, RD, Lori
Valencic, MEd, RD, Nancy Wooldridge, MS, RD, Bonnie A.
Spear, MS, RD

Technical Editor
Michelle L. Kienholz

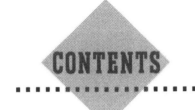

CONTENTS

Introduction

INTRODUCTION

People are talking more and more about sports nutrition for children. This growing interest is an outgrowth of two trends. Health professionals are encouraging America's children to become more physically active, and childhood sports are becoming more competitive. This book, *Play Hard, Eat Right,* deals with common concerns of coaches and parents about nutrition needs of exercising children 6 to 12 years of age.

Children, whether athletes or nonathletes, have dietary needs that are different from those of adults. This book reviews these needs together with issues of growth, development, and body composition. In addition to the basics, we discuss the role of specific nutrients, particularly the major nutrients: carbohydrate, protein, and fat. Other topics include fluids, vitamins, and minerals. We give practical advice on meals before and after competition, training diets, and selecting appropriate foods while traveling. Finally, we deal with more serious issues that have become increasingly prevalent in the United States, such as eating disorders and proper ways to manage weight.

Before beginning the book, please take a moment to review the Young Athlete's Bill of Rights. Child athletes have the right to enjoy their activities and to strive for success. They cannot do so if they hear fallacies or have already formed wrong ideas about how much and what to eat before, during, and after exercise. The information in this book will help ensure that young athletes are guaranteed these rights with regard to proper nutrition for training and competition.

Young Athlete's Bill of Rights

■ ■ ■ ■ ■ ■ ■ ■ ■ ■ ■ ■ ■

All young athletes shall have . . .

The right to
have the opportunity to participate in sports
regardless of ability level.

The right to
participate at a level commensurate with the child's
developmental level.

The right to
have qualified adult leadership.

The right to
participate in a safe and healthy environment.

The right to
share leadership and decision making.

The right to
play as a child and not as an adult.

The right to
proper preparation for participation in sports.

The right to
equal opportunity to strive for success.

The right to
be treated with dignity by all involved.

The right to
have fun through sports.

American Journal of Diseases of Children, 1988; volume 142, page 143.
Reprinted with permission from the American Medical Association.

CHAPTER 1

THE GROWING CHILD ATHLETE

Many coaches and parents have questions about their athletes' growth and development, such as:

- Should 7-year-old boys and girls play soccer together?
- Can my 8-year-old son build his muscles by weight lifting?
- Should my 11-year-old daughter, who has not started to menstruate, try to reduce her body fat?
- How much should my 6 year old weigh?

This chapter answers these and other questions that you might have about children's growth and development. You should be sure that your school-age athletes are growing "on schedule" and that they are eating the right types and amounts of food for their age groups.

You might also need to be careful about how you look at any young "superstars." You may know the importance of body composition—the amount of body fat and muscle mass—in adult athletes. However, because children grow in rapid but somewhat unpredictable spurts, you cannot use ordinary methods for measuring body composition in developing children. Their body chemistry, bone density, and proportion of body water all differ significantly from those of mature athletes, even if their physical performance seems well beyond their years.

1

Physical Growth
■■■■■■■■■■■■

From age 2 until puberty (when children begin to mature sexually), boys and girls grow at about the same rate. You should expect children to grow 2 to 3 inches and gain 3 to 6 pounds each year. There is no physical reason to assign young children to single-sex athletic teams. In fact, many organized sports combine girls and boys in group athletics until age 9 or 10, after which they are separated for social reasons.

At puberty, however, children undergo hormonal changes that mark the beginning of adolescence. These hormonal changes cause them to grow rapidly; therefore, you need to watch children entering puberty very carefully to ensure that they are meeting their nutrition needs. Both boys and girls gain body fat just prior to their growth spurt. By storing extra fat, the body has enough calories to fuel the rapid change in height. You should explain this in advance to growing children so they do not hurt their bodies or stunt their growth by trying to imitate the dieting behavior of adult athletes.

To help monitor child athletes, scientists have devised a numerical system to describe children according to the physical and sexual changes in their bodies. This system is known as the Tanner Stages of Development or Sexual Maturity Ratings.

Although formal Tanner staging is measured by a physician, other characteristics can be used to estimate a child's level of sexual maturity. For a girl, if you know when she menstruated for the first time, you have a good milestone. Between Tanner stages 2 and 3 (usually ages 11 to 12 in the United States), girls undergo their peak growth spurt, with an average gain of 3.25 inches in height. Menstruation begins at stage 4. Once a girl has begun menstruating, she has completed her rapid growth period.

■ ■ ■ ■ ■ ■ ■ ■ ■

Tanner Stages of Development

Stage	Boys	Girls
1.	Before puberty	Before puberty
2.	First appearance of pubic hair	First appearance of pubic hair
	Growth of genitals	Development of genitals
	Increased activity of sweat glands	Increased activity of sweat glands
3.	Pubic hair extends to scrotum	Pubic hair thicker, coarser, curly
	Growth and pigmentation of genitals	Breasts enlarge and pigmentation continues
	Voice changes	Genitals well developed
	Beginning of acne	Beginning of acne
4.	Pubic hair thickens, facial hair begins	Pubic hair abundant, armpit hair begins
	Growth and pigmentation of genitals	Genitals assume adult structure
	Voice deepens	Breasts enlarge and mature
	Acne may be severe	Acne may be severe
		Menstruation begins
5.	Increased distribution of hair	Increased pubic hair distribution
	Genitals fully mature	Breasts fully mature
	Acne may persist and increase	Increased severity of acne (if present)

Peak growth spurt in girls

Peak growth spurt in boys

■ ■ ■ ■ ■ ■ ■ ■ ■

3

Boys grow fastest between Tanner stages 3 and 4 (usually between ages 13 and 14). Boys can expect to grow 8 inches during this phase. Following the growth spurt (in Tanner stage 4), a boy has enough circulating male hormones in his blood to add muscle mass and to show signs of facial hair. If a boy has only "peach fuzz" for facial hair, he may not have completed his growth spurt. The growth spurt lasts much longer in boys than in girls, and after the growth spurt, boys continue to grow at a slow pace until approximately age 20.

Strength

Girls and boys have about the same strength until puberty. Girls gain strength as they grow until they menstruate for the first time. On the other hand, boys continue to become stronger after they finish their growth spurt. After puberty, boys are generally stronger than girls.

By using the Tanner staging system, you can estimate the athletic capabilities of children and teens. Then you can match boys and girls fairly and train them properly. For example:

- A 10-year-old tennis player would benefit very little from a weight-lifting program, because he lacks androgens, the male hormones necessary for muscle development.

- A short 12-year-old basketball player might want to know if she is still in her growth spurt. If she hasn't started to menstruate, the answer is, "Yes."

- An 11-year-old girl should not diet to reduce body fat if she hasn't menstruated for the first time. Her body stores fat just prior to menarche.

Body Measurements
■ ■ ■ ■ ■ ■ ■ ■ ■ ■ ■ ■

Health professionals can check height/weight relationships in children against national growth standards prepared by the National Center of Health Statistics. Physicians and registered dietitians regularly use these charts to assess children's height and weight up to age 18. If you have any question about a child's growth, you should consult with a physician and a registered dietitian.

You may have read about measuring body fat in adult athletes. This practice has become popular in schools and training rooms. A common technique for measuring body fat is underwater weighing, a complicated and expensive method in which the athlete is submerged in a water tank. Bioelectrical impedance, another technique, is not appropriate to use with children because its reliability has been unpredictable. Another method, skinfold measurements with calipers, must be performed by a well-trained professional.

> ■ ■ ■
>
> **Body fat measurements should never be used to manipulate any child's weight for sports competition or to set weight management guidelines. The normal growth and development of the child athlete always must be the primary concern.**

However, measuring fat in children is more difficult because of changes that occur in their bodies before they mature and as they mature. Even trained scientists or health professionals have difficulty accurately estimating the percentage of body fat in children. Special mathematical equations are required. An untrained person who is not familiar with how to take precise measurements will probably overestimate body fat in children and may underestimate lean body weight. These inaccurate estimates could lead to an inappropriate or unsafe weight goal.

Body fat measurements should never be used to manipulate any child's weight for sports competition or to set guidelines for managing his/her weight. A child's normal growth and development always must be the primary concern.

Dietary Recommendations
■ ■ ■ ■ ■ ■ ■ ■ ■ ■ ■

What should young athletes eat? The US Department of Agriculture and Department of Health and Human Services publish the Dietary Guidelines, which recommend a healthful way for all Americans to eat. The Guidelines call for moderation and variety in the diet. The basic rules are:

- Eat a variety of foods.

- Maintain a healthy weight.

- Choose a diet low in fat, saturated fat, and cholesterol.

- Choose a diet with plenty of vegetables, fruits, and grain products.

- Use sugars only in moderation.

- Use salt and sodium only in moderation.

To understand what these guidelines really mean in a child's diet, let us look at the Food Guide Pyramid. Developed by the US Department of Agriculture, the pyramid is a visual guide for planning healthful meals. Each section of the pyramid represents a food category and gives a range for the number of recommended servings to be eaten daily. Most active children (ages 6 to 12) will get the nutrients and energy they need if they eat the number of servings recommended in each layer of the Food Guide Pyramid.

You can help determine whether a child is eating enough calories by tracking his or her height and weight and asking a health professional to compare them with national growth standards. You also should watch how well a child performs and ask whether he or she is tired or "out of steam." If so, he or she may not be eating enough. Of course, a physician or registered dietitian must decide whether the child's diet needs to be changed. If a health professional recommends that your child gain or lose weight, read chapter 9 for general guidelines.

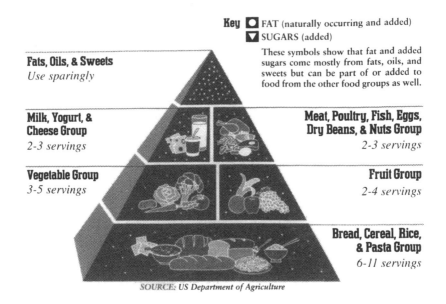

Key ◻ FAT (naturally occurring and added)
▼ SUGARS (added)

Fats, Oils, & Sweets
Use sparingly

These symbols show that fat and added sugars come mostly from fats, oils, and sweets but can be part of or added to food from the other food groups as well.

Milk, Yogurt, & Cheese Group
2-3 servings

Meat, Poultry, Fish, Eggs, Dry Beans, & Nuts Group
2-3 servings

Vegetable Group
3-5 servings

Fruit Group
2-4 servings

Bread, Cereal, Rice, & Pasta Group
6-11 servings

SOURCE: US Department of Agriculture

How Many Servings of Each Food Group Does the Active Child Need Each Day?

Food Group	No. of Servings
Bread	9
Vegetable	4
Fruit	3
Milk	2-3
Meat	2-3

Caloric level is about 2200. The exercising child may need an additional 500 to 1500 calories each day, depending on the frequency, intensity, and duration of physical activity.

■ ■ ■ ■ ■ ■ ■ ■ ■

But before anyone recommends changes in a young athlete's diet, his or her current diet must be examined. Measuring exactly what a child eats is difficult, but a registered dietitian can estimate the amounts of calories, protein, carbohydrate, fat, and vitamins and minerals the child eats on a regular basis. If you are ever concerned about the adequacy of a child's diet, consult a registered dietitian to identify any problems that may be hindering performance.

■ ■ ■ ■ ■ ■ ■ ■

How Big Is a Serving?

Group	Examples
Bread	1 slice of bread or 1/2 bun or bagel 1 ounce of ready-to-eat cereal 1/2 cup of cooked cereal, rice, or pasta
Vegetable	1 cup of raw, leafy vegetables 1/2 cup of chopped, cooked or canned vegetables 3/4 cup of vegetable juice
Fruit	1 medium apple, banana, orange 1/2 cup of cooked or canned fruit 3/4 cup of fruit juice
Milk	1 cup of milk or yogurt 1 1/2 ounces of natural cheese 2 ounces of processed cheese
Meat	2-3 ounces of cooked, lean meat, poultry, or fish 1/2 cup cooked dry beans or 1 egg* 2 tablespoons of peanut butter*

■ ■ ■ ■ ■ ■ ■ ■

Equals 1 ounce of meat.

The most common tools for assessing dietary intake include food records, 24-hour food recalls, and food frequency forms. Samples of these tools for assessing dietary intake are included with this book. If you and your child are interested in keeping records, it is not neccessary to use all of the forms. Review the forms and decide which one best suits your needs depending on the amount of detail you want to include. Some of the forms are more work than others! However, they can be a very helpful starting point when consulting with a registered dietitian regarding your child's diet. Information recorded on a typical food record includes:

- the type or brand of food;
- the amount of food eaten;
- the time at which each food was eaten; and
- the manner in which the food was cooked and/or prepared (including toppings).

Any side effects the food may have had on the athlete during exercise also should be recorded. For example, keeping food records may help a rising track star understand that breakfast cannot be skipped too often, that potato chips eaten before practice do not settle well, or that ice cream eaten in the evening should give way to low-fat frozen yogurt.

Summary

When planning nutrition for a growing athlete, consider the child as well as the sport. You can use his or her stage of growth and development to help predict his or her nutrition needs and physical capabilities. Remember, too, that children look up to coaches, trainers, teachers, and parents as role models. If you set a good example by exercising and eating a nourishing, balanced diet, a child athlete is more likely to "eat to compete" and thereby grow into a healthy adult.

CHAPTER 2

ALL ABOUT CARBOHYDRATE

Young, growing athletes work hard, play hard, and place extra demands on their bodies as a result. Proper training, combined with sound nutrition practices, can help child athletes meet these demands and learn healthy habits for the rest of their lives. However, most children (and adults) neglect nutrition as a key component of good health and athletic performance.

Children, especially in the years before puberty, often skip breakfast and eat the same foods day after day. These habits leave important nutrients out of their diets and may impair growth and athletic performance. Child athletes often need to eat extra calories (see chapter 1), which should be given mainly as carbohydrate foods. This chapter discusses carbohydrate as the preferred fuel for exercise, including the types, sources, and dietary recommendations.

Types of Carbohydrates

Carbohydrate foods, or "carbos," are recognized as the cornerstone of the athlete's diet. Carbohydrate comes mainly from plant foods in two forms, simple and complex.

- *Simple* carbohydrate or simple sugar is sweet. It is easily digested and absorbed into the bloodstream to provide quick energy. Simple carbohydrate is found in milk, fruits, and sugary products (candy, cookies, soda).

- *Complex* carbohydrate is starchy. Starches found in vegetables like potatoes and corn are examples. They provide energy more slowly, because they take longer to be digested into sugar and to be absorbed into the bloodstream as glucose. Complex carbohydrate is also found in breads, cereals, pasta, rice, and other starchy foods.

Which is Better?

- Both simple and complex carbohydrates provide energy to working muscles.

- Foods high in complex carbohydrate contain more essential nutrients, such as B vitamins, iron, dietary fiber, and minerals.

- Simple carbohydrate, especially from foods such as candy and soft drinks, may provide energy but it lacks essential vitamins and minerals.

- Most carbohydrate in the diet should be obtained from complex carbohydrate food sources.

Carbohydrate in Exercise

After the body digests carbohydrate, it uses it to provide energy. For immediate energy, carbohydrate is turned into glucose, which is circulated in the blood. The liver and muscles can store carbohydrate as glycogen, which can be used for energy (as glucose) later during exercise.

The body uses carbohydrate mainly to provide energy for the muscles to do work. How much and what type of fuel (glucose or fat) is used depends on how intense the activity is and how long the exercise lasts.

- Brief, intense exercise, such as sprinting or weight lifting, uses glucose from glycogen stored in the muscles for fuel.

- Intermittent sports, such as basketball or football, also use glucose from stored glycogen for fuel.

- Endurance sports, such as long-distance running or cycling, use glycogen stores first and then turn to body fat (see chapter 4) for energy.

- For any activity, the body prefers to use carbohydrate for energy.

However, the muscles and liver can store only a limited amount of glycogen. Athletes must replace glycogen by eating more carbohydrate, especially after exercise. Child athletes who experience fatigue or sluggishness might be training too hard, might be dehydrated, might be eating too little, or might be eating too little carbohydrate. Active children should eat 50 to 55 percent of their total calories in the form of carbohydrate.

Dietary Recommendations
■ ■ ■ ■ ■ ■ ■ ■ ■ ■ ■ ■

Young athletes should think of carbohydrate when they think about food. For example, the child athlete who needs 2500 calories per day would need to eat at least 313 to 343 grams of carbohydrate (there are 4 calories per gram of carbohydrate). Foods that have high levels of complex carbohydrate, such as potatoes, rice, cereals, and starchy vegetables, are excellent sources of glucose as well. Fruits, fruit juices, and dairy products contain natural simple sugars. Review the following list of high-carbohydrate foods to make suggestions to your young athletes.

13

■ ■ ■ ■ ■ ■ ■ ■ ■

High-Carbohydrate Foods

Bread, Cereal, Rice, and Pasta

These foods provide a higher percentage of complex carbohydrate.

	Serving	Energy (calories)	Carbohydrates (grams)
Bagel	1/2	83	16
Biscuit (2" across)	1	103	13
Blueberry muffin	1	110	17
Bread (white,whole-wheat)	1 slice	61	12
Bread sticks	2 sticks	77	15
Bun (hot dog, hamburger)	1/2	60	11
Cereal	1 oz. (1 c.)	110	24
Cereal (cooked Cream of Wheat®)	1/2 c.	64	13
Corn bread (2" square)	1/2 piece	89	14
English muffin	1/2	77	15
Graham crackers	2 squares	60	11
Noodles (spaghetti)	1/2 c. cooked	80	17
Oatmeal (cooked)	1/2 c.	73	13
Oatmeal (flav. instant)	1 packet	110	25
Pancakes (4" across)	1	56	9
Popcorn (plain)	1 c. popped	26	6
Pretzels	1 oz.	106	21
Rice (brown)	1/2 c. cooked	116	25
Rice (white)	1/2 c. cooked	112	25
Saltines	5 crackers	60	10
Tortilla (flour)	1	85	15
Waffles (3 1/2" across)	1	60	9

Other baked goods

These foods provide both complex and simple carbohydrate.

	Serving	Energy (calories)	Carbohydrates (grams)
Angel food cake	1 piece	142	32
Animal crackers	5	56	10
Chocolate cake	1 piece	235	40
Fig bar	1	50	10
Granola bar	1	109	16
Oatmeal raisin cookie	1	62	9

Combination foods

These foods provide a higher percentage of complex carbohydrate.

	Serving	Energy (calories)	Carbohydrates (grams)
Bean burrito	1	393	32
Pizza (cheese)	1 slice	290	39

Fruits

These foods provide a higher percentage of simple carbohydrate.

	Serving	Energy (calories)	Carbohydrates (grams)
Apple	1 med.	81	21
Apple juice	3/4 c.	83	21
Applesauce	1/2 c.	116	30
Banana	1	105	27
Cantaloupe	1/2 c.	29	7
Cherries (raw)	10	49	11

Fruits continued

	Serving	Energy (calories)	Carbohydrates (grams)
Dates (dried)	5	114	30
Fruit cocktail (packed in own juice)	1/2 c.	56	15
Grape juice	3/4 c.	72	17
Grapes	1/2 c.	74	19
Orange	1 med.	65	16
Orange juice	3/4 c.	84	20
Pear	1	77	19
Pineapple	1/2 c.	39	10
Prunes (dried)	5	100	26
Raisins (seedless)	1/3 c.	151	39
Raspberries	1/2 c.	31	7
Strawberries	1/2 c.	23	6
Watermelon	1/2 c.	25	6

Vegetables

These foods provide a higher percentage of complex carbohydrate.

	Serving	Energy (calories)	Carbohydrates (grams)
Carrot	1 med.	31	8
Corn	1/2 c.	89	21
Lima beans	1/2 c. cooked	109	20
Peas (green)	1/2 c.	63	12
Potato (baked, plain)	1 large	220	50
Sweet potato	1 large	118	28

Milk, Yogurt, and Cheese

These foods provide a higher percentage of simple carbohydrate.

	Serving	Energy (calories)	Carbohydrates (grams)
Frozen yogurt (low-fat)	1 c.	220	34
Fruit flavored yogurt	1 c.	225	42
Milk (1%)	1 c.	121	12
Milk (skim)	1 c.	86	12
Pudding	1/2 c.	161	30

■ ■ ■ ■ ■ ■ ■ ■ ■

Depending on their need for calories, child athletes can add more carbohydrate to their diets by eating at least the following amounts from the Food Guide Pyramid groups:

- Six servings from the Bread, Cereal, Rice, and Pasta Group
- Three servings from the Milk, Yogurt, and Cheese Group
- Three servings from the Vegetable Group
- Two servings from the Fruit Group

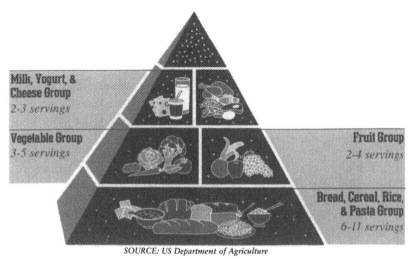

Milk, Yogurt, & Cheese Group
2-3 servings

Vegetable Group
3-5 servings

Fruit Group
2-4 servings

Bread, Cereal, Rice, & Pasta Group
6-11 servings

SOURCE: US Department of Agriculture

17

You can help children remember which foods to choose by putting the the foods on "teams" as shown here. Ask your children to pick winning carbohydrates from each team to eat.

■ ■ ■ ■ ■ ■ ■ ■ ■

Winning Carbohydrates

Bread, Cereal, Rice, and Pasta Team	*Fruit and Vegetable Team*	*Milk, Yogurt, Cheese Team*
Bagels	Apples	Milk
Breads	Bananas	Yogurt
Cereals	Broccoli	Pudding
Crackers	Corn	Frozen yogurt
English muffins	Carrots	Sherbet
Graham crackers	Fruit juices	
Pancakes	Nectarines	
Pasta (spaghetti, macaroni)	Oranges	
Popcorn	Pears	
Potato, sweet potato	Peas	
Pretzels	Peppers (green, red)	
Rice	Tomatoes	

■ ■ ■ ■ ■ ■ ■ ■ ■

The sample menu that follows would be appropriate for many young athletes and would provide about 2500 calories. About 55 percent of calories would come from carbohydrate, 15 to 20 percent from protein, and 25 to 30 percent from fat.

Providing well-balanced meals and snacks for child athletes can be a challenge. To help children eat more carbohydrate, you can:

■ Encourage them to eat carbohydrate-rich foods at meals and as snacks.

- Include at least one serving each from the Bread, Cereal, Rice, and Pasta Group; the Vegetable Group; the Fruit Group; and the Milk, Yogurt, and Cheese Group at each meal. (Two-thirds of the food on children's plates should have plenty of carbohydrate!)

- Pack easy-to-carry carbohydrate foods for lunch and pre-practice snacks: bagels, oatmeal raisin cookies, fruit bars, pretzels, fig bars, low-fat yogurt, popcorn, fresh fruit or juice, pudding, raisins, bananas, and so forth.

- Let young athletes have a "refreshment" break during practice to drink fluids and to eat carbohydrate-rich snacks.

- Correct poor eating habits gradually by including more nutritious foods.

- Encourage children to help make their own meals and snacks.

- Serve children's favorite foods along with nutritious, high-carbohydrate, low-fat foods.

■ ■ ■ ■ ■ ■ ■ ■ ■

Sample Menu

Meal	Menu
Breakfast	2 pancakes Syrup 1 cup 2% milk
Snack	1 bagel Jam or jelly 6 ounces orange juice
Lunch	1 slice vegetable pizza Carrot and celery sticks 2 graham crackers 1 cup 2% milk

Sample menu continued

      Snack (Before practice)
            2 fig bars
            16 ounces water

      Snack (After practice)
            1 box fruit juice
            1 packet raisins

Dinner   3 ounces roasted chicken breast
            1/2 cup rice
            1 slice bread
            Lettuce and tomato
            1 tablespoon dressing
            1 cup 2% milk

Snack   1 cup frozen yogurt
            1 cup lemonade
            1 sandwich-
               2 slices multigrain bread,
               3 ounces lean turkey,
               lettuce, tomato,
               and mustard

Summary

In general, child athletes need more energy to fuel both their exercise and their normal growth and development. Eating carbohydrate allows the muscles to store glycogen for fuel during exercise. Children who do not eat enough carbohydrate may not train or compete up to par. You should encourage all school-age children—particularly child athletes—to eat more carbohydrate foods and to replace high-fat items, such as chips, ice cream, and pastries, with more healthful, high-carbohydrate foods, such as breads, corn, fruits, and spaghetti.

CHAPTER 3

ALL ABOUT PROTEIN

Protein is an essential part of child athletes' diet . . . as long as the child eats it in moderation. The role of protein in sports nutrition has reached mythical proportions that must be reduced to reality. What is the real story? The following common questions about protein will be answered here:

- How does the body use protein?

- Will extra protein improve an athlete's performance?

- How much protein does the child athlete need?

Athletes can adjust the amount of protein they eat for optimal performance in training and in competition. However, protein and *amino acids* (which make up protein) have no magical qualities that guarantee success. Protein alone cannot and will not improve athletic ability, no matter what manufacturers of special amino acid supplements want the public to believe. This chapter addresses dietary protein and protein needs for young athletes.

Protein in the Body
■ ■ ■ ■ ■ ■ ■ ■ ■ ■ ■ ■

Protein is one of the basic nutrients found in most foods. It is made from building blocks called amino acids. Although some advertisements suggest that certain amino acids build muscle, amino acids actually build protein that the body uses in many different ways. Despite the many claims that protein boosts athletic performance, the main function of protein is to maintain and repair all body tissues. Protein also makes:

- hemoglobin, which takes oxygen to all cells.

- antibodies, which fight off infection and disease.

- enzymes and hormones, which regulate body functions.

Eating more than the recommended amount of protein does not improve any of these functions, and it does not make stronger or larger muscles. Extra protein is usually stored as fat, not as muscle. As a result, eating too much protein can sometimes hurt the body more than it helps it.

Building Muscles
■ ■ ■ ■ ■ ■ ■ ■ ■ ■ ■ ■

The body uses protein to make muscle tissue, but eating large amounts of protein does not lead to the development of larger, stronger muscles. Muscles do not get bigger unless the body has enough male hormones (androgens) in the blood (see chapter 1). Boys and girls both add muscle during puberty, but boys eventually have more androgens circulating in the bloodstream, which result in greater muscle mass. Even these androgens do not magically build muscles. To gain muscle mass, athletes must increase the workload on their muscles (with training) and eat a balanced diet that contains adequate calories.

How Much Protein Should Young Athletes Eat?

■ ■ ■ ■ ■ ■ ■ ■ ■ ■ ■ ■

Although the Recommended Dietary Allowances (RDAs) tell you how much protein boys and girls should eat at different ages, you should consider other factors:

- *Maturity*—Young athletes may have slightly higher protein needs if they are at or beyond a certain stage of sexual maturity. The key question is whether or not they have the proper hormones for adding muscle mass (see chapter 1 for discussion of the maturation process).

- *Carbohydrates*—Although it is not recommended, young athletes who eat little carbohydrate may need slightly more protein. If children eat the recommended high-carbohydrate diet, they should need only the recommended amount of protein for their age and sex.

- *Calories*—Young athletes who eat too few calories may need slightly more protein. However, the best idea would be to increase overall food intake.

- *Training*—Young athletes who follow hard, exhausting training schedules may need more protein, but only during the training season.

- *Protein sources*—Young athletes who eat most or all of their proteins from plant sources must be careful to eat a wide variety of grains and vegetables. Meanwhile, children who eat proteins from a variety of animal sources (meat, milk, eggs) usually do not have to worry about getting enough protein.

Most children 6 to 10 years old need to eat about 0.5 gram of protein per pound of body weight each day. Young athletes who might need slightly more protein (for reasons previously described) can eat 0.6 to 0.9 gram of protein per pound of body weight. You should realize, though, that this additional amount of protein is supplied in just an extra glass of milk or an extra serving of meat (3 to 4 ounces).

■ ■ ■ ■ ■ ■ ■ ■ ■

Recommended Daily Allowances (RDAs) for Protein

Age (years)	Gender	Daily Protein Intake (grams)
4-6	boys and girls	24
7-10	boys and girls	28
11-14	boys	45
15-18	boys	59
11-14	girls	46
15-18	girls	44

■ ■ ■ ■ ■ ■ ■ ■ ■

For example, your 10-year-old soccer player should eat about 0.5 gram of protein per pound of body weight. If he weighs 70 pounds, he should eat about 35 grams of protein per day. If your soccer player needs slightly more protein because of the reasons discussed in this chapter, he or she should eat no more than 0.6 to 0.9 gram of protein per pound of body weight per day. The 70-pound soccer player, therefore, should not eat more than 42 to 63 grams of protein per day, even during rigorous training.

Protein in Foods
■■■■■■■■■■■■

Young athletes can easily meet their protein needs with a diet that includes at least the following amounts of foods recommended in the Food Guide Pyramid:

- Two to three servings of meat, poultry, fish, dry beans and peas, eggs, nuts
- Three servings of low-fat milk, yogurt, cheese, pudding
- Six servings of bread, cereal, rice, pasta
- Three servings of vegetables

Young athletes should spread their protein choices throughout the day, rather than having one large serving of protein-rich food in the evening. They also should eat a variety of protein foods from each of the food groups.

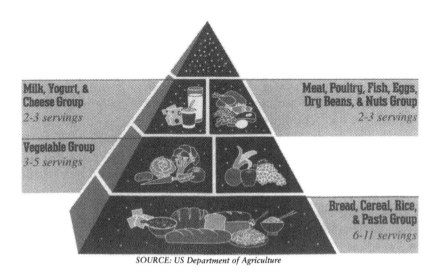

SOURCE: US Department of Agriculture

■ ■ ■ ■ ■ ■ ■ ■ ■

Protein in Various Foods

Food	Protein (grams)	Serving Size
Milk	8	8 oz. (1 c.)
Yogurt	8	8 oz. (1 c.)
Cheese	13	2 oz. (processed)
Fish	21	3 oz. (tuna sandwich)
Poultry	21	3 oz. (grilled chicken sandwich)
Meat (beef)	21	3 oz. (hamburger, roast beef sandwich)
Peanut butter	8	2 Tbsp.
Nuts	5-7	1 oz. (1 handful)
Eggs	7	1

■ ■ ■ ■ ■ ■ ■ ■ ■

What About Protein Supplements?
■ ■ ■ ■ ■ ■ ■ ■ ■ ■ ■ ■

Protein, whether from food or dietary supplements, is made up of amino acids. While some amino acids can be made in the body, others cannot. The ones that are made in the body are called nonessential amino acids. The ones that are not made in the body are called essential amino acids and must be eaten in the diet. Of the 22 amino acids, 13 are nonessential and 9 are essential.

■ ■ ■

Amino acid supplements do not improve athletic performance, and they do not increase muscle size or strength.

If you think that a young player may need any type of nutritional supplement, please reconsider. One of the dangers of eating too much protein is dehydration. Protein and amino acid supplements are especially

26

unnecessary in children, since most supplements contain no more protein or amino acids than are found in a serving of meat or a glass of milk. And supplements are expensive. The body treats amino acids from powders the same way as it does amino acids from oat cereal.

■ ■ ■ ■ ■ ■ ■ ■ ■

Amino Acids Provided in Food Source Versus Supplement

Amino Acid	Quantity (milligrams) in Cereal (1 oz.) + Milk (1/2 cup)	Quantity (milligrams) in Amino Acid Supplement*
Threonine (essential)	329	24
Isoleucine (essential)	588	40
Lysine (essential)	492	135
Methionine (essential)	171	20
Cysteine (nonessential)	144	0
Phenylalanine (essential)	425	280
Tyrosine (nonessential)	346	8
Valine (essential)	519	8
Arginine (nonessential)	465	1000
Histidine (essential)	205	0

*This is an average "amino acid package."

■ ■ ■ ■ ■ ■ ■ ■ ■

Vegetarian Diet
■ ■ ■ ■ ■ ■ ■ ■ ■ ■ ■ ■

When recommending how much protein to eat, health professionals generally assume that the athlete will consume a variety of foods from all food groups—meat, milk, bread, vegetable, and fruit. Animal foods—such as eggs, milk, yogurt, cheese, fish, poultry, beef, and pork—contain proteins that include all the essential amino acids.

Proteins found in plant products (vegetables and grains) are "incomplete," meaning that they do not contain all nine essential amino acids. Therefore, vegetarian athletes must eat a wide variety of plant proteins to ensure a combination of all essential amino acids. Plant foods that lack one or more amino acids can be eaten with other plant foods that are rich in the missing amino acid(s). The table below shows examples of how you can eat a combination of plant foods to get all the essential amino acids.

■ ■ ■ ■ ■ ■ ■ ■ ■

Plant Food Combinations Yielding
All Essential Amino Acids

Rice + beans (kidney, pinto, lima, navy)

Croutons + split-pea soup

Tortillas + beans

Corn bread + chili beans

Brown bread + baked beans

Whole-wheat bread + peanut butter

Tofu + sesame seeds

■ ■ ■ ■ ■ ■ ■ ■ ■

A young athlete who follows a vegetarian diet must be careful of what he or she eats. The vegetarian diet can be nutritionally complete so long as a wide variety of foods are consumed over the course of a day. However, any child on a vegetarian diet should consult with a registered dietitian to check the nutritional adequacy of his or her diet. The dietitian can teach the young athlete and his or her parents about a balanced vegetarian diet.

Also, the dietitian may advise the child to eat milk foods and eggs to make sure that he or she grows properly and can remain physically active. A vegetarian who does not eat animal flesh, eggs, or milk products may be at risk for nutrient deficiencies of:

- Vitamin B12—found reliably only in animal sources and in some fortified cereals.

- Calcium—best consumed in milk, yogurt, and other dairy products.

- Iron—not absorbed as well from plant sources as from animal sources. Even a small portion of meat, poultry, or fish with an iron-rich vegetable will help the body absorb iron.

Eliminating foods that contain important vitamins and minerals can make healthful eating more of a challenge. If you do this, you and your child must be prepared to take on the added responsibility necessary to maintain good health and proper growth.

Summary

Protein is essential to the overall health, growth, and development of child athletes. It should come from low-fat animal sources and/or from a wide variety of plant foods. High-protein diets are unnecessary for any athlete—especially child athletes—since most Americans usually consume more protein than their bodies need. Eating excessive amounts of protein burdens the body, which stores the excess protein as fat. Unfortunately, athletes of all ages continue to use protein and amino acid pills, powders, and drinks in the hope of increasing muscle mass and strength. Remember, the advertisements for "body-building" supplements promote false hopes of increasing muscle mass when the only actual increase is in the companies' profits!

CHAPTER 4

ALL ABOUT FAT

The body needs a certain amount of fat to maintain its normal functions. Dieting to gain or lose body fat can have dramatic effects on the body during critical stages of growth. Consequently, health professionals discourage children from dieting to gain or lose body fat when their weights are in the normal range, as discussed in chapter 1. Body fat comes mainly from fat in the diet, though excessive amounts of protein and carbohydrate can be stored as fat as well. This chapter provides guidelines for how much fat exercising children should eat and discusses the amount of fat in various foods.

Fat in the Body

Fats and oils are essential nutrients in the human diet. You can add fat (such as margarine or oil) to foods to enhance flavor, thus encouraging finicky eaters to eat a wider variety of foods. For example, adding margarine to corn may improve the taste for the child who might not eat it otherwise. When athletes eat fat in moderation, it can be a concentrated source of energy.

Fat in the diet:

- supplies more than twice as much energy as protein and carbohydrate (9 calories per gram of fat compared to 4 calories per gram of carbohydrate or protein).

- helps the body absorb and use certain vitamins (A, D, E, and K, which are fat-soluble vitamins).

- supplies essential fatty acids that the body needs to survive.

The body stores fat beneath the skin, around the organs, and inside the muscles. Sometimes the muscles use fat as a fuel in the form of triglycerides, which are present in food and are also made in the liver and intestines. Triglycerides are made of fatty acids (individual fat units) that determine whether fat is saturated, polyunsaturated, or monounsaturated. Saturated fats (such as butter or beef fat) are less healthy, particularly for the heart, than unsaturated fats (such as safflower and corn oil) and monounsaturated fats (such as olive and peanut oil).

Fat in Exercise
■ ■ ■ ■ ■ ■ ■ ■ ■ ■ ■

As we said earlier, blood sugar and muscle glycogen give working muscles most of their energy. The following factors determine how much fat the body uses for energy:

- Duration of exercise—The body uses fat tissue to provide energy, but you must exercise for 30 minutes before enough fatty acids are available for fuel. Until then, carbohydrate (glycogen) provides most of the energy.

- Intensity of exercise—As the intensity of the exercise increases, working muscles have less oxygen available to burn fat. During sports that have short bursts of very intense activity, such as a 200-yard dash, a 50-yard swim, or a baseball game, the body burns very little fat for energy.

Fat in the Diet
■ ■ ■ ■ ■ ■ ■ ■ ■ ■ ■ ■

How much fat should your young athletes eat? Fat stores play an important role in athletic performance, and fat is an essential nutrient for a growing child. Young athletes must take extra care to eat enough calories, protein, and essential vitamins and minerals so the added stress of athletic activity does not affect his or her growth. When helping a young athlete plan his or her meals, you must consider the recommended percentage of calories from fat, safe levels of cholesterol, and preferred food sources.

The typical American diet supplies almost 40 percent of total calories as fat. This figure is too high and may be responsible for the high incidence of many chronic diseases (such as heart disease, cancer, and diabetes). The American Dietetic Association, the American Academy of Pediatrics, the US Department of Health and Human Services' National Cholesterol Education Program, the American Heart Association, and the National Cancer Institute support the following guidelines for fat consumption:

■ ■ ■

These recommendations do not apply to infants from birth to 2 years of age. Infants need to eat a higher percentage of fat calories because they grow so fast.

- Total fat—No more than 30 percent of total daily calories

- Saturated fat—Less than 10 percent of total daily calories

- Cholesterol—Less than 300 milligrams per day

The Food Guide Pyramid recommends using fats and oils sparingly in the diet. You should eat foods that are low in saturated fat, low in total fat, and low in cholesterol. You should also choose a variety of foods. This strategy helps you eat enough carbohydrate, protein, and other nutrients while eating only enough calories to maintain desirable body weight.

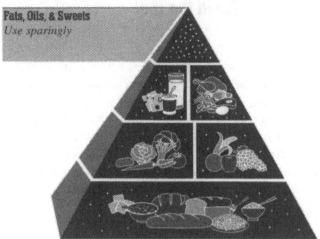

Fats, Oils, & Sweets
Use sparingly

SOURCE: *US Department of Agriculture*

To determine the amount of fat in a child's diet, you may want to examine recent food records with a registered dietitian (see chapter 1 and forms provided in this book). They can be used to estimate how many calories the child is eating and to identify any high-fat foods in the diet. Because most food labels provide the fat content in terms of grams, you may find it easier to calculate the number of fat grams that can be eaten each day. Divide caloric intake by 30 to determine the number of fat grams that will provide 30 percent of calories as fat. For example:

- 2000 calories ÷ 30 = 67 grams of fat (30 percent of calories)

- 2200 calories ÷ 30 = 73 grams of fat (30 percent of calories)

- 2400 calories ÷ 30 = 80 grams of fat (30 percent of calories)

Note that this holds true only for 30 percent. Do not divide by a different number, such as 28, to calculate the number of fat grams for 28 percent of calories from fat.

Most people should be concerned about reducing the amount of fat they eat. The key to achieving this in child athletes' diets is moderation. You should not be too strict or too liberal with fat.

Taking too much fat out of the diet also can take the fun out of eating. Children, especially physically active children, need a lot of energy and, therefore, need to eat moderate amounts of fat. Of course, children who eat a lot of fried foods, snack foods, desserts, or fast foods (see chapter 8) are probably consuming too much fat. The excess fat may be replacing other essential nutrients.

Cholesterol in the Diet

■ ■ ■ ■ ■ ■ ■ ■ ■ ■ ■

Cholesterol is found only in animal products. Usually foods that have a lot of cholesterol also have a lot of saturated fat—but not always. For example, shellfish (such as shrimp) are very low in saturated fat but relatively high in cholesterol. However, it is always better to select the low-fat shellfish over the high-fat meat. Eating foods that are high in saturated fat raises blood cholesterol levels more than eating foods that are high in cholesterol. The National Cholesterol Education Program recommends that adults, as well as healthy children and teens, eat no more than 300 milligrams of cholesterol per day.

Summary

■ ■ ■ ■ ■ ■ ■ ■ ■ ■ ■

The best training diet supplies the athlete's body with all the essential nutrients in the right amounts. Fat is a concentrated source of energy that also makes food taste better. If nutritious foods taste better, your young athlete is more likely to eat nutritionally balanced meals. Severely restricting the amount of fat a child can eat to improve fitness can be dangerous. The child loses a critical source of calories. And prolonged fat restriction can have other negative effects on the child's growth and development.

VITAMINS AND MINERALS

With the wide variety of foods and places to eat today, it can be difficult to be sure children are getting all of the essential nutrients. However, you do not need vitamin and mineral supplements to ensure adequate nutrient intake. You easily can give children a well-balanced and enjoyable diet of foods readily available in the supermarket.

Preadolescent children may have slower growth rates and reduced appetites. However, they still must eat enough nutrients to meet minimal dietary requirements and to get ready for their upcoming growth spurt. For young athletes, proper nutrition also promotes optimal athletic performance. Both you and your child athletes should know which convenient, nutrient-dense foods can meet daily requirements and improve performance. You should make a wide variety of these foods easily accessible to children both at home and in school. This chapter reviews the functions and sources of essential vitamins and minerals and discusses their role in child athletes' diets.

How Vitamins Help

The body needs to get vitamins through food since it cannot make them on its own. Vitamins are essential for life, but some can be

37

reused and, therefore, are needed only in very small amounts each day. The fat-soluble vitamins—A, D, E, and K—are stored in the fat tissues of the body. Water-soluble vitamins are not stored in the body and must be replaced every day. These include C, thiamin, riboflavin, B6, niacin, folacin, biotin, and pantothenic acid. The following table gives food choices for two important vitamins—A (fat soluble) and C (water soluble).

■ ■ ■ ■ ■ ■ ■ ■ ■

Food Choices for Vitamins A and C

Vitamin A for healthy growth, skin, and vision	Vitamin C for healthy teeth, bones, and blood vessels	Vitamins A and C
Asparagus	Brussels sprouts	Broccoli
Carrots	Cauliflower	Kale
Collard greens	Okra	Peppers (green, red, chili)
Mixed vegetables	Potatoes	
Mustard greens	Bananas	Spinach
Pumpkin	Grapes	Sweet potatoes
Winter squash (acorn, butternut, etc.)	Grapefruit, grapefruit juice	Tomatoes
Apricots	Peaches	Turnip greens
Cherries (red sour)	Honeydew melon	Cantaloupe
Nectarines	Lemons	Mangoes
Guavas	Oranges, orange juice	Papayas
Prunes	Raspberries	Plums (purple)
Milk	Strawberries	
	Tangerines	
	Tangelos	
	Watermelon	

■ ■ ■ ■ ■ ■ ■ ■ ■

Vitamins have many functions in the body. Most of them help the body use carbohydrate, fat, and protein. Vitamins also are involved in making red blood cells, regulating growth, clotting blood, and maintaining vision. By keeping the body working properly, vitamins help maintain health and, in children, proper growth and development. However, eating more vitamins or eating them more frequently does not enhance any of the functions that might be useful to athletic performance.

Get the Facts

- The best source of vitamins is a healthful, balanced diet.
- Vitamins have not been shown to prevent or cure any disease (including the common cold) except for those related to specific vitamin deficiencies (for example, vitamin C cures scurvy).
- Although some vitamins help the body produce and use energy, they do not provide energy themselves (because they do not contain any calories).
- There is no difference between vitamins made in a laboratory and "natural" vitamins from plants or animals (except "natural" vitamins are usually more expensive).
- Vitamin supplements cannot be used to replace foods or make up for poor dietary habits.
- B15 (pangamic acid) is not a vitamin.
- Taking extra vitamins will not make a child mature faster or become stronger.
- Some vitamins are toxic at high doses. "If a little is good, more must be better" does not apply to any vitamins.

Minerals in the Body
■ ■ ■ ■ ■ ■ ■ ■ ■ ■ ■

Minerals are also essential and perform a variety of functions in the body. Some are used to make specific tissues. For example, calcium and phosphorus are used to build teeth and bones. Others, such as iodine, are used to make hormones. Iron is one of the most important minerals for an athlete because it is a part of hemoglobin, which carries oxygen throughout the body. (Oxygen is needed by working muscles and all tissues.) Minerals also regulate muscle contraction and body fluids, help transmit nerve impulses, and maintain a normal heart rhythm. Minerals are divided into two groups, macrominerals and trace minerals, depending on the body's needs.

■ ■ ■ ■ ■ ■ ■ ■ ■

Mineral Groups

Macrominerals (Body needs more)	Trace Minerals (Body needs less)
Calcium	Iron
Phosphorus	Manganese
Magnesium	Copper
Sodium	Iodine
Potassium	Zinc
Chloride	Cobalt
Sulfur	Fluoride
	Selenium

■ ■ ■ ■ ■ ■ ■ ■ ■

Eating too much of one mineral can interfere with the body's attempt to use another. For example, eating too much phosphorus can lower calcium levels and lead to bone loss; too much zinc

40

can impair copper levels. As with vitamins, eating more minerals does not speed up or improve how minerals work but instead can disturb the body's overall balance. The following two tables give food choices for three important minerals—iron, zinc, and calcium—in the diets of young athletes.

Many complex factors influence the body's absorption of iron. The body absorbs iron in meat more easily than iron from plant sources. Foods that are rich in vitamin C (tomatoes, oranges, melons, lemons, strawberries) may help the body absorb iron from other sources.

■ ■ ■ ■ ■ ■ ■ ■ ■

Sources of Iron and Zinc

Iron *for healthy red blood cells (oxygen to muscles)*	Zinc *for healthy growth and development*	Iron and zinc
Enriched/whole-grain breads, pasta, and cereal	Veal	Dry beans and peas
Beans (green, lima)	Bagels	Beef
Broccoli	Bran muffin	Chicken
Spinach	Oat cereal	Fish
Potato with skin	Raisin bran	Lamb
Tomato juice	Rice	Pork
Winter squash (acorn, butternut, etc.)		Shellfish
Apricots (dried, canned)		Turkey
Prunes		Peas
Raisins		Nuts

■ ■ ■ ■ ■ ■ ■ ■ ■

Nutrient Needs of Athletic Children
■ ■ ■ ■ ■ ■ ■ ■ ■ ■ ■ ■

Athletic children do need some nutrients in higher amounts. Young athletes need extra calories and fluids to support their physical activity. If they eat extra foods to provide enough energy, they usually get any additional vitamins or minerals they may need as well. However, according to scientific studies, athletic activity does not seem to significantly increase vitamin or mineral needs. If your young athletes eat a balanced diet of foods they like, they will get enough of the needed vitamins and minerals. You have lots of food choices for each vitamin and mineral. The table on page 43 shows the wealth of vitamins and minerals that a healthful, balanced diet can supply even for the pickiest eaters.

Spotlight on Calcium
■ ■ ■ ■ ■ ■ ■ ■ ■ ■ ■

Children need at least three servings of calcium-rich foods each day so that:

- bones grow strong and hard
- teeth develop properly

■ ■ ■ ■ ■ ■ ■ ■ ■

Foods belonging to the Calcium Club include:

Milk	Calcium-fortified	Custard
Milk shakes	juices	Frozen yogurt
Pudding	Cheese	Macaroni and
Yogurt	Cheese pizza	cheese
Ice cream	Cream soups	

■ ■ ■ ■ ■ ■ ■ ■ ■

. . . .

Vitamins and Minerals in Commonly Eaten Foods

Food	*Vitamins and Minerals*
Beef, chicken, fish, ham, pork, turkey	Iron, phosphorus, potassium, zinc, niacin, riboflavin, thiamin, vitamins B6 and B12
Peanut butter, almonds, walnuts, peanuts, seeds, other nuts	Copper, magnesium, phosphorus, vitamins A and B12
Black beans, chick-peas, kidney beans, lentils, navy beans, peas, pinto beans, soybeans	Iron, magnesium, phosphorus, potassium, folate
American, cottage, cheddar, part-skim mozzarella, ricotta, Swiss, and other cheese	Calcium, phosphorus, vitamins A and B12
Bagels, corn bread, grits, crackers, pasta, corn muffins, noodles, pita bread, ready-to-eat cereals, white bread, rolls	Iron, thiamin, riboflavin, niacin
Brown rice, corn tortillas, oatmeal, whole-grain rye bread, whole-grain ready-to-eat cereal, whole-wheat pasta, crackers, bread, rolls	Copper, iron, magnesium, phosphorus, thiamin, riboflavin, niacin, vitamin E
Low-fat (1%) milk, low-fat flavored milk, skim milk, buttermilk, 2% milk, whole milk	Calcium, phosphorus, potassium, riboflavin, vitamins A and D (if fortified)
Oranges, grapefruit, cantaloupe, watermelon, strawberries, blueberries, raspberries, tangerines	Potassium, folate, vitamins C and A (if deep yellow)

Vitamins and minerals continued—

Food	*Vitamins and Minerals*
Apples, apricots, bananas, cherries, fruit juice, grapes, peaches, pears, pineapples, plums, prunes, raisins	Potassium, vitamins C and A (if deep yellow)
Broccoli, carrots, green peppers, kale, pumpkin, spinach, sweet potatoes, winter squash	Iron, magnesium, potassium, folate, riboflavin, vitamins A, C, K, E, and B6
Black-eyed beans, corn, lima beans, green peas, potatoes	Iron, magnesium, phosphorus, potassium, folate
Cabbage, cauliflower, celery, cucumbers, green beans, lettuce, onions, summer squash, tomatoes, vegetable juice, zucchini	Magnesium, potassium, folate, vitamins C and K

■■■■■■■■

Dietary Recommendations
■■■■■■■■■■■■

Vitamin and mineral needs can be met easily by eating a well-balanced diet. Achieving such a diet over the long run is of major importance. Nutrient deficiencies develop over months, not days, and a healthy person can adapt to temporary shortages. More is not necessarily better! Young athletes can meet their vitamin and mineral needs with diets that include the foods and servings recommended in the Food Guide Pyramid.

Because children often do not eat enough fruits and vegetables in particular, they may miss out on some important sources of vitamins and minerals. Here are some ideas for helping children eat more fruits and vegetables.

Eating Vegetables Can Be Fun!

■ ■ ■ ■ ■ ■ ■ ■ ■ ■ ■ ■

- Have children choose a vegetable at the grocery store and make it "veggie of the week."
- Have children help plant and harvest a vegetable garden.
- Let children help prepare vegetables for eating (washing, peeling, cooking).
- Try dipping cut vegetables into yogurt, cheese, salsa, or bean dip.
- Instead of serving the same vegetables prepared the same way, try new vegetables in new combinations and new cooking techniques:

—Stir-fry vegetables in a tablespoon of oil with small portions of meat or chicken.

—Add vegetables to chicken noodle soup.

—Lightly steam vegetables that you might normally serve raw.

—Replace carrot and celery sticks with raw cherry tomatoes, sugar-snap peas, green or red pepper strips, cauliflower or broccoli florets, summer squash, radishes, or mushrooms.

—Add chopped green and red pepper to corn.

—Grate carrots and mix with raisins and apple chunks.

—Add chopped raw spinach and red cabbage to lettuce for a colorful salad.

—Sprinkle grated cheese on top of steamed vegetables.

- Offer vegetables at the beginning of a meal when children are hungriest and not filled up on other foods.
- Serve small portions of vegetables cut in a variety of shapes.

New Fruit Combos
■■■■■■■■■■■■

- Make frozen juice pops in an ice cube tray.
- Freeze grapes, strawberries, bananas, and melon balls for frosty summer treats.
- Try serving peaches or apricots with baked chicken or turkey, or add a pineapple slice to a hamburger!
- Introduce children to unfamiliar fruits from other regions or nations, such as papaya, mango, kiwi, and figs.
- Add fruit to gelatin molds.
- Top pound cake or angel food cake with vanilla or lemon yogurt and fruit.
- Select canned fruits packed in light syrup or natural juice rather than in heavy syrup.
- Serve pineapple rings with a cherry in the middle.

Supplements Not Needed
■■■■■■■■■■■■

Many well-meaning parents and coaches advise young athletes to take supplements as health insurance. Giving young athletes supplements can give them a false sense of security and may encourage future supplement use. They may assume that their morning dose of supplements provides them with all the vitamins and minerals they need so they can eat cookies and soda instead of fruit and yogurt.

Another disadvantage to using supplements is that athletes, particularly children, are likely to associate performance gains with whatever supplements they may be taking. Of course, this is not true, but it may make children less willing to attribute gains to training, hard work, and a balanced diet. This type of false reinforcement also may make them try other types of supplements and substances (including, possibly, drugs and steroids). The result may be a snowball effect with undesired consequences. Megadoses of supplements do not make up for lack of training or talent, and they do not give athletes a competitive edge.

To move away from this reliance on "supplement insurance," you must reinforce your young athletes' confidence in regular foods for promoting muscle growth and optimal performance. To further help them resist the pressure to take supplements, you can help children keep records of what they eat, when and how hard they train, and how their athletic performance improves (see page 129). Then you can point to good dietary and training habits as the cause of any improvement, rather than leaving the children to associate good performance arbitrarily with a pill or powder. This approach empowers children to exert control over their athletic performance as well as all areas of their lives.

Summary
■ ■ ■ ■ ■ ■ ■ ■ ■ ■ ■ ■

Vitamins and minerals are substances that the body needs and can receive through a balanced diet. As with a car, overfilling the gas tank does not improve performance. In some cases, eating large amounts of certain vitamins and minerals can be dangerous. Young athletes should concentrate on eating a variety of foods to meet their vitamin and mineral needs.

CHAPTER 6

THE IMPORTANCE OF FLUIDS

You might be surprised to learn that the most important part of any athlete's diet is fluids. While humans can survive for about a month without food, they can only survive a few days without water. Athletes need to drink extra fluids to replace body water lost while exercising. Child athletes must be especially careful to drink enough fluids while exercising. The type, amount, timing, and even the temperature of fluids consumed can affect how well the body replaces its fluids. As a coach or parent, you are responsible for preventing heat disorders in exercising children, and you must make sure that they drink enough fluids. This chapter will help you deal with the special needs of younger athletes in maintaining proper body water levels.

Special Fluid Needs of Children

Compared with adults, or even teenagers, preadolescent children need to be especially careful about drinking enough water for many reasons:

- Children do not handle temperature extremes well.
- Children sweat less.

- Children get hotter during exercise.

- Children's hearts have a lower output of blood.

- Children have more skin surface for their body weight.

All these factors increase the risk of dehydration for children. Therefore, fluids play a critical role in maintaining the health and optimal performance of your child athlete. In addition, conditions in some sports make it necessary for athletes to pay particular attention to body water levels.

- Football and hockey players wear protective gear, which reduces the ability of the body to cool itself.

- Swimmers often do not realize that they lose body water through sweat. They also can become dehydrated by sitting around in a hot, humid environment between sessions.

- Athletes in sports that have weight categories for competition (such as wrestling) should never deprive themselves of food, or especially water, to lose weight.

How Fluids Cool the Body
■ ■ ■ ■ ■ ■ ■ ■ ■ ■

One of the most important functions of water is to cool the body. As a child exercises, working muscles generate heat, and this raises the temperature of the entire body. When the body gets hot, it sweats, and as the sweat evaporates, the body is cooled. If the child does not replace this sweat by drinking more fluids, the body's water balance will be upset, and the body may overheat.

> ■ ■ ■
> Give your young athletes personalized water bottles containing cold water and tell them to drink 3 to 4 oz. every 15 minutes.

Humid days require even more care. If the air is humid, sweat does not evaporate, and the body is not cooled. This can lead to overheating and heat disorders that may require medical attention.

How Much Water is Enough?

■ ■ ■ ■ ■ ■ ■ ■ ■ ■ ■

All athletes must drink water before, during, and after exercise. Dehydration can start when an athlete loses as little as 1 percent of body weight. In a 70-pound child, this would be less than 1 pound of weight loss. Young athletes should be weighed before they train or compete and again during the event (if it will be especially long) or afterwards so you know how much water they have lost. Follow the basic guidelines below to be sure that a child is drinking enough water throughout an exercise session.

■ ■ ■ ■ ■ ■ ■ ■ ■

Guidelines for Drinking Water

Before Exercise	*During Exercise*	*After Exercise*
Drink 10 to 14 oz. of cold water 1 to 2 hours before the activity.	Drink 3 to 4 oz. of cold water every 15 minutes.	Drink 2 cups (16 oz.) of cold water for every pound of weight loss.
Drink 10 oz. of cold water or diluted fruit juice 10 to 15 minutes before the activity.		

■ ■ ■ ■ ■ ■ ■ ■ ■

You must watch and see how much water a young athlete actually drinks. Supervision is essential because children do not instinctively drink enough fluid to replace body water losses. Thirst does not indicate when an athlete needs more fluids. The body's thirst mechanism does not work well during exercise, and the athlete constantly must be reminded to drink. Children may not recognize the symptoms of heat strain, and they may push themselves to the point of heat injury.

Choosing the Right Fluids
■ ■ ■ ■ ■ ■ ■ ■ ■ ■ ■

Plain, cold water is the best and most economical source of fluid. The body absorbs cold fluids faster than warmer ones, and drinking water is the easiest way to replace body fluids. Young athletes also can use sports drinks, especially during activities lasting more than 90 minutes. These drinks should contain between 6 and 8 percent carbohydrate or 15 to 18 grams of carbohydrate per cup. If products labeled "sports drinks" do not meet these guidelines, they may need to be diluted.

Water is adequate for most children. However, some are more likely to drink sufficient amounts if you give them flavored fluids. Sports drinks or diluted fruit juice are appropriate choices. Be sure to dilute fruit juice at least twofold: 1 cup of water for every 1 cup of juice. Tell children not to drink carbonated sodas or undiluted fruit juice as a fluid source during exercise. These beverages are too rich in carbohydrate (which can cause stomach cramps, nausea, and diarrhea). Caffeinated beverages (such as tea, coffee, and cola beverages) will dehydrate the body even more.

Athletes can also replace their body fluids with foods containing a lot of water, such as oranges, watermelon, apples, grapes, lettuce, and tomatoes, along with water. These foods provide water and carbohydrate, and they are good for replacing lost water and lost energy (glycogen) after exercise.

Salt Tablets
■ ■ ■ ■ ■ ■ ■ ■ ■ ■ ■

The recommendation here is simple: *Athletes should never take salt tablets.*

Salt tablets contribute to dehydration because they cause extra water to enter the stomach and draw it away from other body tissues. They also irritate the stomach lining and can cause nausea.

You may have heard that inadequate salt intake causes muscle cramps, but they are more likely caused by larger losses of water through excessive sweating. You should realize that sweat contains more water than sodium and potassium (electrolytes). The priority for any athlete should be to replace body water, not salt. Children will replace any electrolytes that they might have lost after exercise just by eating a healthful diet. Fruits and fruit juices are excellent sources of electrolytes.

Again, never give salt tablets to children. They do not help performance, but they do increase the risk for heat disorders and injury.

Dehydration and Heat Disorders

Dehydration is the loss of body fluid. If allowed to continue, this fluid loss not only affects athletic performance, it also becomes life-threatening. Exercising without drinking fluids dehydrates the body by itself. The body becomes dehydrated even faster under the following conditions:

- *Temperature*—The higher the temperature, the greater the sweat losses.

- *Humidity*—The higher the relative humidity, the greater the sweat losses.

- *Intensity of Exercise*—The harder the athlete works, the greater the sweat losses. A twofold increase in speed produces a fourfold increase in sweat!

- *Body Size*—The larger the athlete, the greater the sweat losses (boys generally sweat more than girls).

- *Duration of Exercise*—The longer the workout, the greater the sweat losses.

- *Fitness*—Well-trained athletes sweat more, and they start sweating at a lower body temperature. Remember, the function of sweating is to cool the body, and the well-trained body cools more efficiently.

As water is lost during exercise, the body experiences a progression of heat-related illnesses. In addition to weighing young athletes before and after workouts and giving them personalized water bottles to drink from throughout exercise sessions, you must watch for the symptoms of heat disorders and take appropriate action immediately.

■ ■ ■ ■ ■ ■ ■ ■ ■

Heat Disorders

Symptoms	*Disorder*	*Treatment*
Thirst Chills Clammy skin Throbbing heart Muscle pain Spasms Nausea	Heat cramps	Have the child drink 4 to 8 oz. of cold water every 10 to 15 minutes. Move the child to the shade and remove any excess clothing.
Reduced sweating Dizziness Headache Shortness of breath Weak, rapid pulse Lack of saliva Extreme fatigue	Heat exhaustion	Move the child to a cool place. Have the child drink 16 oz. (2 c.) of water for every pound of weight lost. Remove wet clothes and put ice behind the child's head.
Lack of sweat Lack of urine Dry, hot skin Swollen tongue Visual disturbances Rapid pulse Unsteady gait Fainting Low blood pressure Loss of consciousness Shock	Heat stroke	Call for emergency treatment. Place ice on the back of the child's head. Remove wet clothing. If conscious, help the child take a cold shower. If in shock, elevate feet.

Preventing Heat Disorders
■ ■ ■ ■ ■ ■ ■ ■ ■ ■ ■ ■

In addition to making sure that your young athletes drink enough fluids, you can take a number of precautions to reduce the risk of heat injury.

- Schedule workouts for the coolest times of the day (before 10 a.m. or after 6 p.m.), particularly in warmer climates. Note the humidity and wind as well.

- Allow children to adjust to warmer conditions gradually. Restrict the length and intensity of training sessions for the first 4 to 5 days and then increase the intensity slowly for another 1 to 2 weeks.

- Avoid excessive clothing, taping, or padding on hot or humid days. You can help improve body cooling by having the children change from sweaty clothes to dry ones. They also should wear white or light-colored clothing made of lightweight cotton or mesh material and low-cut socks.

- Schedule breaks in the shade or other shelter. This will allow the children's bodies to cool down from the heat that built up during exercise.

- Never use water restrictions as a disciplinary measure. Water—preferably chilled water—must be available at all times during training and competition.

- Make sure that each child comes to practice or competition fully hydrated. Remind everyone in advance about how much water to drink before arriving.

- Weigh children before and throughout exercise to identify the ones who lose weight during practice or competition.

- Schedule water breaks during which all children must drink a minimum amount of water. Be especially strict with those who previously lost large amounts of weight during workouts.

- Pay close attention to children who are at risk for heat disorders due to obesity, poor conditioning, weight loss during exercise, or other health problems.

- Discourage the deliberate practice of dehydration. Tell young athletes that it keeps them from performing up to par athletically and can hurt their bodies seriously.

- Adjust the timing of practice and competition (time of day, season of year) as needed to prevent heat disorders. Extreme heat and/or humidity are valid reasons to cancel a scheduled workout or competition.

You should decide whether to modify or even cancel practice based on the air temperature and humidity, which can be measured with a wet bulb thermometer available at hardware stores. Here are specific guidelines for deciding whether to reduce exercise intensity or to cancel it altogether:

—If the wet bulb temperature is below 66° F, no precautions are necessary. Watch closely children who are susceptible to heat disorders.

—When the temperature is 66° F to 78° F, be cautious. Insist that unlimited amounts of water (preferably iced) be given, and monitor athletes closely for symptoms of heat disorders.

—Wet bulb temperatures above 78° F mean real danger for serious heat disorders. You must keep practice light, modifying or eliminating some routines as needed, and allow the athletes to work out in minimal gear. Water breaks in the shade are mandatory. Children who lose weight during exercise should not participate.

—The precautions previously described also must be followed if the relative humidity is 95 percent or higher, regardless of the wet bulb reading.

Summary
■ ■ ■ ■ ■ ■ ■ ■ ■ ■ ■ ■ ■

Coaches, trainers, and parents must supervise young athletes closely, making sure that they drink enough fluids to avoid dehydration. Heat stroke ranks second among reported causes of death in high school athletes. Weighing children before and after exercise is the best way to check whether they are drinking enough fluids to replace losses. In addition to stressing adequate fluid intake, you must educate young athletes about the danger of extreme weight-loss practices that severely dehydrate the body.

CHAPTER 7

PRE- AND POST- EVENT MEALS

Before exercise, the time when child athletes eat is as important as what they eat. Of course, foods eaten routinely affect health and sports performance more than anything eaten the day of the event. As we said in chapter 2, all athletes should eat most of their calories in the form of carbohydrate to store enough energy as glycogen. However, food eaten before, during, and after practice and competition can dramatically affect how an athlete feels while exercising. An upset stomach on game day usually results from poor food choices that morning. This chapter will help you plan appropriate pre- and post-event and training meals for your young athlete.

Pre-Event Meals

The pre-event meal serves two main purposes: first, to prevent athletes from feeling hungry before or during the event, and second, to help supply fuel to the muscles during training and competition. Still, most of the energy needed for any sports event is provided by whatever the athletes have eaten during the prior week. The best plan for the pre-event meal is to provide foods that children like and that contain lots of carbohydrate, low to moderate amounts of protein, and even less fat. Keep in mind the following guidelines:

- High-fat and high-protein foods take longer to digest than carbohydrate foods. If an athlete eats high-fat or high-protein foods a few hours before exercise, he or she risks having indigestion, nausea, and vomiting during exercise.

- To have a relatively empty stomach while exercising, the child should eat no sooner than 1 to 3 hours before practice or competition.

- Eating sugary foods such as candy and honey right before exercise does not provide quick energy.

Athletes should avoid eating simple carbohydrate (such as sugar, honey, candy, or soft drinks) for quick energy before exercise. Most of the energy for exercise comes from foods eaten several hours and days prior to the start of the event. Additionally, some athletes are more sensitive than others to changes in blood glucose levels when they eat simple sugars. Athletes should check their sensitivity to these changes by eating different amounts and sources of carbohydrate before exercising.

■ ■ ■ ■ ■ ■ ■ ■ ■

Eating Before the Event

1 to 2 Hours Before	2 to 3 Hours Before	3 or More Hours Before
Fruit or vegetable juice	Fruit or vegetable juice	Fruit or vegetable juice
Fresh fruit (low fiber, such as plums, melon, cherries, peaches)	Fresh fruit	Fresh fruit
	Breads, bagels	Breads, bagels
	English muffins	English muffins
	No margarine or cream cheese	Peanut butter, lean meat, low-fat cheese
		Low-fat yogurt
		Baked potato
		Cereal with low-fat (1%) milk
		Pasta with tomato sauce

■ ■ ■ ■ ■ ■ ■ ■ ■ ■ ■

Sample Meals (3 to 4 Hours Before the Event)

A.M.

1 c. orange juice
Bagel
2 Tbsp. peanut butter
2 Tbsp. honey

or

1 c. orange juice
3/4 c. corn flakes
Medium banana
Wheat toast and jelly
1 c. low-fat milk

or

1 c. orange juice
Pancakes and syrup
English muffin and jelly
1 c. low-fat yogurt

or

1 c. orange juice
Waffles and strawberries
1 c. low-fat yogurt

P.M.

1 c. vegetable soup
2 oz. skinless chicken
2 slices wheat bread
2 slices tomato
1 c. low-fat frozen yogurt
1 c. apple juice

or

Large baked potato
1 tsp. margarine
Carrot sticks
1/2 c. fruit salad
1 c. low-fat milk

or

Salad:
    lettuce, 1 oz. ham,
    1 oz. turkey, 2 slices
    tomato, carrot sticks,
    2 Tbsp. dressing
1/2 cup pudding

or

2 c. spaghetti
2/3 c. tomato sauce with
    mushrooms
French bread
1 c. lemon sherbet
1 c. low-fat milk

■ ■ ■ ■ ■ ■ ■ ■ ■ ■ ■

Your young athlete can choose from many good sources of complex carbohydrate to eat before exercise. You can offer him or her breads, pastas, rice, cereals, pancakes, rolls, bagels, English muffins, tortillas, fruits (bananas, apples, oranges), and vegetables (corn, peas, potatoes). These foods are all digested quickly so the athlete's stomach is empty and blood sugar level is stable by the time the practice or competition begins. Foods that are rich in carbohydrate also help to replenish energy (glycogen) stores, which athletes may need during prolonged training or competition. Refer to the table on page 61 for suggestions on what to eat before exercising.

Sometimes children are too nervous or excited to eat on the day of an event. In this case, offer water and juice. However, in most cases, you should be able to follow these simple pre-event guidelines.

■ ■ ■ ■ ■ ■ ■ ■ ■

Pre-Event Reminders

Eat	Avoid Large Amounts
Complex carbohydrate	Fat
Water	Protein
Moderate portions	Fiber
3 to 4 hours before event	Last-minute sweets

■ ■ ■ ■ ■ ■ ■ ■ ■

Eating at All-Day Events
■ ■ ■ ■ ■ ■ ■ ■ ■ ■ ■ ■

During all-day competition or training, carbohydrate foods and drinks may delay the onset of fatigue. However, you may have difficulty finding nutritious food choices at regional tournaments, such as track, swimming, soccer, basketball, tennis, volleyball, or wrestling. If possible, bring snacks for the team. Otherwise, children need to make wise choices at concession stands or bring snacks from home.

The "Instead of" foods listed below will stay in the stomach longer and impair performance. Drinking plenty of fluids is important. In general, water is adequate, but the flavor of sports drinks may encourage children to drink more fluids. Just be sure that the carbohydrate level is not too concentrated (no more than 6 to 8 percent, or 15 to 18 grams of carbohydrate per cup).

■ ■ ■ ■ ■ ■ ■ ■ ■

If You're Going to Compete

Try	*Instead of . . .*
Bagels	Candy bars
Bananas	Doughnuts
Fruit juice	French fries
Muffins	Hot dogs
Pretzels (hard or soft)	Nachos/Potato chips
Sports drinks (6 to 8% carbohydrate)	Soda

■ ■ ■ ■ ■ ■ ■ ■ ■

Post-Event Meals
■ ■ ■ ■ ■ ■ ■ ■ ■ ■ ■ ■

As soon as children stop exercising, give them water and fruit juices to replace body fluids. Also give them complex carbohydrate sources to replenish their glycogen stores. The body is most efficient at absorbing and storing energy (glycogen) during the first 4 to 5 hours after exercise. In fact, the post-event meal is probably more important than the pre-event meal because it determines how much energy an athlete will have for the next training session or competition. Immediately after training or competing, your young athlete should choose from the following foods and drinks:

- Medium bagel (50 grams carbohydrate)
- Pretzels (23 grams carbohydrate per 1 ounce)
- Fruit yogurt (40 grams carbohydrate per 8 ounces)
- Large banana (40 grams carbohydrate)
- Cranberry-apple juice (43 grams carbohydrate per 8 ounces)
- Apple juice (30 grams carbohydrate per 8 ounces)
- Orange juice (28 grams carbohydrate per 8 ounces)

About 2 hours after exercising, child athletes should eat a meal that contains mostly carbohydrate: yogurt and fruit, cheese and bagel, vegetable pizza, or spaghetti and meat sauce. You can follow the guidelines given for pre-event meals and include more protein and fat.

Summary

■ ■ ■ ■ ■ ■ ■ ■ ■ ■ ■ ■

What and when an athlete eats on game day is important. Child athletes should learn early the healthful and scientific way to improve performance through diet. This early education can prevent them from developing superstitious and potentially harmful routines on their own. As with the daily diet, the emphasis in the athlete's game day diet should be carbohydrate (especially complex carbohydrate) foods prior to and after training and competing. You might think that a quick snack just before lining up should give athletes an extra boost, but it may, in fact, slow them down. The post-event meal is important for restoring energy to athletes' muscles. The basic rules for eating before and after exercise are simple, easy to follow, and not mysterious or magical.

CHAPTER 8

MEALS ON THE GO

Americans are eating more and more of their meals on the go. A 1990 Gallup survey found that Americans eat out an average of 3.7 times per week. Until recently, few nutritious, balanced food choices were available in fast-food restaurants. In the past few years, however, fast-food franchises and family-style restaurants began to take healthful eating seriously, and they added more low-fat foods to their menus. Now, convenience foods can be nutritious and can fit in any budget. This chapter offers simple guidelines for making healthful food choices away from home.

Fast Food

Many coaches and parents choose convenience foods for child athletes because of tight time schedules. Although the amount of time available may seem to outweigh nutrition considerations, the two need not conflict. Fast-food establishments provide quick service, inexpensive meals, and consistent food quality at easily accessible locations. Although many fast foods still have too much fat and salt and not enough vitamins, minerals, and fiber, many franchises now offer low-fat, nutritious food choices as well.

When stopping at a fast-food restaurant, remember to focus on finding low-fat, high-carbohydrate foods. Be sure to be a role model yourself! Check the following table on fast-food meal plans to learn what meals to "go for."

■ ■ ■ ■ ■ ■ ■ ■ ■

Fast-Food Meal Plan

Go For It!	*Stop and Think Again!*
Pancakes with syrup Low-fat (1%) milk Orange juice	Biscuit with egg, cheese, and bacon Whole milk
Baked potato with chili Roll with 1 pat margarine Garden salad with 1/4 packet dressing Low-fat yogurt milkshake	Hot dog with chili and cheese Onion rings Chocolate malt
Thick-crust vegetable pizza Bread sticks Garden salad, 1 ladle dressing Low-fat (1%) milk	Double cheese, double pepperoni pizza Fried mozzarella cheese Regular soda
Single hamburger Muffin Orange juice	Deluxe double cheeseburger Large French fries Regular soda Apple pie or turnover

■ ■ ■ ■ ■ ■ ■ ■ ■

Family-Style Restaurants

■ ■ ■ ■ ■ ■ ■ ■ ■ ■ ■ ■

Family-style restaurants offer a wider variety of nutritionally sound choices than do fast-food restaurants. Eating a meal together before or after a game or competition can be an enjoyable experience for children, parents, and coaches. Once again, remember that children learn good dining habits by watching adults select healthful food items.

Breakfast items, such as pancakes, cereal, bagels, and English muffins, are an inexpensive and easy way to select high-carbohydrate meals. Children enjoy many other menu items that also offer sound sports nutrition. Check the lunch or dinner menus listed below and consider why they would or would not be good for athletes in training.

■ ■ ■ ■ ■ ■ ■ ■

Family-Style Restaurant Meal Plans

Go For It!	*Stop and Think Again!*
Roast beef sandwich (lettuce and tomato)	Fried fish with tartar sauce
Fruit juice	Onion rings
Low-fat vanilla milkshake	Soda
Spaghetti with tomato sauce	Crispy fried chicken
Bread with 1 pat margatine	Mashed potatoes with butter and gravy
Garden salad, 1 ladle dressing	Biscuits with butter
Fruit cup	Whole milk
Low-fat (1%) milk	

■ ■ ■ ■ ■ ■ ■ ■ ■

Grocery and Convenience Stores
■■■■■■■■■■■■

Where can you buy food for the young athlete at an all-day soc-cer tournament? Grocery stores, convenience stores, and conces-sion stands are usually the choices available. Unfortunately, they typically tempt customers with high-fat, non-nutritious foods. Shoppers often overlook grocery and convenience stores as sources of quick, inexpensive, nutritious snacks and meals. With guidance from coaches and parents, young athletes can choose fruits, juices, muffins, and low-fat dairy products rather than candy bars, snack chips, and soft drinks. Make looking for snacks fun! Ask a child to find something good to drink (low-fat milk, juice, water), and then ask him or her to scout for a food that is creamy, crunchy, or juicy.

■■■■■■■■■

Grocery Store Snack Suggestions

Creamy	*Crunchy*	*Juicy*
Banana	Apple	Berries
Low-fat cheese	Carrots	Oranges
Peanut butter	Cereal	Peaches
Pudding	Crackers	Plums
Yogurt	Popcorn	Watermelon
	Pretzels	

■■■■■■■■■

Sometimes event organizers will honor requests for specific food items, for example, fruit juice, fruit, and bread products. If the host of the tournament or race does not plan to offer nutrition-ally sound foods, be sure to bring a cooler of high-performance snacks or to locate a nearby source of low-fat, high-carbohy-drate foods.

Summary

■ ■ ■ ■ ■ ■ ■ ■ ■ ■ ■

Providing young athletes with food guidelines will help them to pick out high-performance foods from almost any menu or food aisle. Diets that are high in carbohydrate and fluids, moderate in protein, and low in fat will give child athletes enough calories and nutrients to grow, train, and compete. It takes practice to find such high-performance choices at fast-food establishments, family-style restaurants, and grocery stores, but it can be done. Usually you can request brochures that provide nutrition information from fast-food franchises. If the restaurant manager does not have any in the store, he or she can give you the address to write to for more information.

Of course, it is also important to let kids be kids. An occasional ice cream cone, candy bar, or bag of chips is completely acceptable. However, kids should eat them occasionally in addition to high-performance foods, not in place of them!

CHAPTER 9

BODY WEIGHT AND THE CHILD ATHLETE

Is there really an "ideal" body weight for competition? Some people believe that reaching a certain body weight will make a child more competitive. Attaining a "competitive" weight may mean gaining or losing weight for an imagined competitive edge. However, as the child progresses in a sport, he or she may develop compulsive eating behaviors and become obsessed with reaching and maintaining a specific "competitive" weight. Add the irregular eating schedules, meal skipping, and excessive snacking common among all children, and the potential for problems begins to snowball.

More than ever, children are experimenting with fad diets, diet pills, and weight-gain powders and pills, all of which are dangerous to growing bodies. Such extreme eating behaviors also can lead to eating disorders, such as anorexia nervosa and bulimia nervosa. Determining whether a child needs to gain or lose weight and then deciding how to do it is quite a challenge and should never be undertaken without supervision by a physician and a registered dietitian. This chapter addresses the issues of reaching a "competitive" weight and reviews appropriate methods for gaining or losing weight. It also discusses the early signs, symptoms, and approaches for dealing with disordered eating behaviors.

71

Losing Fat

■■■■■■■■■■■

You have probably seen it happen. As competition day approaches, a young athlete may panic, feeling that he or she is too fat to win. In some cases it may be true, but the days and even weeks prior to competition are the worst times to start trying to lose weight. A starved athlete may not perform effectively, and one who has attempted an unsafe weight-loss method will be even more disadvantaged. As we said in chapter 1, young children need a certain amount of food calories that provide energy to grow normally.

Some young athletes experiment with diuretics, starvation or fad diets, or other methods to lose weight quickly. Rapid weight loss usually rids the body of water weight and possibly even lean body tissue from muscles or vital organs. For any athlete, these methods lead to dehydration, low muscle glycogen stores, fatigue, and poor performance. For the still-growing child athlete, the risks are even greater. Check the following table for some tips on working with an overweight child.

Working With an Overweight Child

■■■■■■■■■■■

Parents

- Consult with a registered dietitian if you think your child might have a weight problem.
- Do not single out the overweight child in your family by serving "special foods" or imposing restrictions.
- Encourage the overweight child to eat slowly and to enjoy whatever he or she eats.
- Never give food as a reward or withhold it as a punishment.

- Be a role model: exercise and eat a balanced, low-fat diet yourself.
- Do not tell a child that he or she is "on a diet."

Coaches

- Do not single out the overweight child by making him or her run extra laps or exercise longer.
- Never restrict fluids for any child.
- Never refer to a child as fat, obese, or overweight, especially in front of his or her teammates.
- Watch for signs of heat distress. Overweight children are at higher risk for heat disorders than thinner children.
- Be patient!
- Be a role model: eat a balanced diet, keep active, and maintain a healthy body weight.

Many children will attain their goal weights simply by changing their diets and exercising more. A good strategy is to replace high-calorie, high-fat foods with nutritious, low-calorie, high-carbohydrate foods. This approach improves athletic performance, produces some weight loss, and helps steer children toward a healthy lifestyle. As a result, they can gradually "grow into" their weight. However, when the physician and registered dietitian recommend weight or fat loss, diet alone is not an effective method for reducing body fat. Exercise is also important. The following guidelines will help young athletes lose weight gradually and safely.

Setting goals

- Only health-care experts, such as physicians and registered dietitians, should recommend a specific body weight as a goal. They can consider the child's level of sexual maturity, growth, and development. Many times the child athlete may not need to lose weight but instead needs to grow to a height that is appropriate for his or her weight.

- Weight loss goals must be realistic and achievable—usually not more than 10 percent of body weight at a time. Otherwise, a child could become frustrated, particularly if he or she has trouble keeping the weight off later.

- The child should reach the goal weight at least 3 to 4 weeks prior to the start of training and competition. This will help him or her participate at peak performance.

- Cut back on foods that provide empty calories (for example, sodas, candy bars, chips, cookies), and emphasize low-fat foods from the food groups featured in the Food Guide Pyramid.

Less energy in (eat less)

+

more energy out (exercise more)

=

fat loss

- Weight loss should be slow—no more than 1/2 pound per week (depending on age and weight).

- Exercise more often for longer periods, but only at moderate intensity (heart rate of about 130 beats per minute).

- Do aerobic exercise, such as fast walking, running, hiking, biking, swimming, or other continuous rigorous activity.

- Choose family activities that include exercise. Excessive television watching—even if the entire family is present—can affect children's eating habits.

Television and Weight Control

—For the entire family, discourage eating meals or snacks while watching television.

—Watch television with children. Discuss advertisements and how they can be misleading.

—Be selective about what children watch on television. Limit the time they spend in front of the television or playing video games.

Specific Strategies
■ ■ ■ ■ ■ ■ ■ ■ ■ ■ ■ ■

- Eat 3 servings of low-fat milk products (1 serving = 8 ounces of milk or yogurt, or 1 1/2 to 2 ounces cheese).

- Eat 2 to 3 servings of lean meats, poultry, or fish (1 serving = 2 to 3 ounces cooked lean meat).

- Eat 2 to 4 or more servings of fruits (1 serving = 1 medium fruit, 1/2 cup chopped, or 3/4 cup juice).

- Eat 3 to 5 servings of vegetables (not fried, no added sauces, no butter or margarine; 1 serving = 1/2 cup cooked or raw, 3/4 cup of juice).

- Eat 6 to 11 servings of breads, cereals, pasta, rice, or other grains (skip pastries; 1 serving = 1 slice of bread, 1/2 cup cooked cereal, rice, or pasta, or 1 ounce of ready-to-eat cereal).

- Eat at regular intervals—3 meals plus planned snacks—to avoid hunger and impulse eating. Check the table on page 76 for a sample weight control menu for one day.

- Stick to a planned exercise schedule that includes 3 to 5 aerobic workouts per week that last more than 30 minutes.

■ ■ ■ ■ ■ ■ ■ ■ ■

Sample Menu for Weight Control

Breakfast 3/4 c. orange juice
3/4 c. raisin bran (1 tsp. sugar optional)
1 slice whole-wheat toast
1 Tbsp. jam or jelly
1 c. low-fat (1%) milk

Lunch 1 turkey sandwich—
3 oz. turkey breast
2 slices whole-wheat bread
mustard
sliced tomato and lettuce
1 apple
1 c. low-fat (1%) milk

Snack 1 banana

Dinner 3 oz. lean beef
1 medium baked potato
1/2 c. plain nonfat yogurt
1/2 c. green beans
1 c. low-fat (1%) milk
1/2 c. ice milk

Snack 3/4 c. tomato juice
1 oz. pretzels
1/4 c. raisins

■ ■ ■ ■ ■ ■ ■ ■ ■

Gaining Weight
■■■■■■■■■■■■

Gaining weight can give too-thin child athletes the competitive edge to win. To gain weight, children must consume more calories than they use for growth and exercise. They also must continue to exercise to prevent gaining weight as fat, rather than as muscle. Of course, as we said in chapter 1, only children who have reached puberty have the hormones to build larger, stronger muscles. For example, boys who are too young to add muscle mass should not eat more protein foods in an attempt to "bulk up" for sports like football or hockey.

Extra calories should come mainly from additional carbohydrate. Protein intake should remain at levels recommended for the athlete's age and sex. Athletes should adjust their fat intake only to continue eating 30 percent of their calories as fat. The following guidelines will help young athletes gain weight appropriately.

Setting Goals
■■■■■■■■■■■■■

- Goals must be realistic, particularly because children already require a lot of food. Eating even more to gain weight may be difficult.

- Only health-care experts, such as physicians and registered dietitians, should recommend a specific body weight as a goal. They can consider the child's level of sexual maturity, growth, and development.

- Gaining weight slowly and steadily means adding less body fat and more lean body weight, or muscle. No more than 1/2 pound should be gained each week (depending on age and weight).

- Children who train at a competitive level may need to eat as many as 3,000 to 4,000 calories every day to gain weight.

More food in
(change in diet)

+

muscle use
(exercise)

=

lean body weight gain

- Children should increase portion sizes and eat more snacks between meals to gain weight. Or they can eat smaller amounts more often (5 to 6 small meals) throughout the day.

- Children who eat to gain weight should take care not to eat too much fat (particularly saturated fat) and cholesterol.

- Adolescents can use weight-training exercises that work muscles hard to add bulk and strength while gaining weight.

Specific Strategies

- Eat a large bedtime snack that includes food from all food groups (for example, a peanut butter and banana sandwich with low-fat milk).

- Eat foods with plenty of complex and simple carbohydrates (for example, pancakes and syrup, orange juice, low-fat milk, pizza, and low-fat milk shakes). Check the table on page 79 for a sample day's menu for gaining weight.

- Use weight-gain supplements only if your physician or registered dietitian recommends them. Drinks are expensive, but sometimes it is easier to drink 500 calories than to eat them. One suggestion is a powdered breakfast mix made with low-fat milk. Snack bars are also expensive and usually provide no more calories than a store-bought breakfast or granola bar eaten with a glass of low-fat milk. Powders are very expensive and usually are made just of egg white solids, soy protein or dry milk, and a carbohydrate source.

■ ■ ■ ■ ■ ■ ■ ■ ■

Sample Menu for Weight Gain

Breakfast

1 c. orange juice
6 pancakes
1/4 c. syrup
2 pats margarine
1 1/2 c. low-fat (1%) milk

Snack

1 soft pretzel
1 1/2 c. tomato juice

Lunch

1 turkey sandwich—
    4-5 oz. turkey breast
    1 7-in. pita bread pocket
    2 Tbsp. light mayonnaise
    chopped tomato and lettuce
1 c. fruit yogurt
2 c. apple juice
1 large muffin

Snack

1 package powdered breakfast mix
1 c. low-fat (1%) milk

Dinner

1 medium vegetable-cheese pizza
2 c. low-fat (1%) milk
1/4 c. raisins

Snack

1 peanut butter and jelly sandwich—
    3 Tbsp. peanut butter
    3 Tbsp. jelly
    2 slices whole-grain bread
1 c. low-fat (1%) milk

■ ■ ■ ■ ■ ■ ■ ■ ■

Eating Disorders Among Athletes

■ ■ ■ ■ ■ ■ ■ ■ ■ ■ ■ ■

Some athletes try to become thin at any cost. Often one of those costs is the development of an eating disorder. Disordered eating behaviors may be triggered by many factors:

- crash dieting

- intense desire for athletic success

- fear of failure

- a seemingly harmless comment by a coach or parent about the athlete's weight

- frustration or guilt about not being able to control body weight

Children often continue inappropriate dieting rituals into adulthood. Consequently, you must teach young athletes early in their careers about the dangers of eating disorders and about healthy methods for controlling their weight. Look over the lists of warning signs for two major eating disorders—anorexia nervosa and bulimia nervosa—so that you can recognize potential problems in your young athletes. Note, however, that the presence of just one or two of these symptoms does not necessarily indicate the presence of an eating disorder. Appropriate health professionals—a physician, registered dietitian, or psychologist—should always see the child involved before anyone makes a diagnosis.

■ ■ ■ ■ ■ ■ ■ ■ ■

Eating Disorders

Anorexia Nervosa

Sudden, large weight loss
Preoccupation with food, calories, and weight
Wears baggy or layered clothing
Relentless, excessive exercise
Mood swings
Avoids food-related social activities

Bulimia Nervosa

Noticeable weight loss or gain
Excessive concern about weight
Visits bathroom after meals
Depressive moods
Strict dieting followed by eating binges
Increasingly criticizes his or her body

■ ■ ■ ■ ■ ■ ■ ■ ■

Coaching Your Athlete

■ ■ ■ ■ ■ ■ ■ ■ ■ ■ ■

As a coach or parent, you can dramatically influence the eating and exercise behaviors of young athletes. Be careful about what you say, especially about body size. Strong athletes are better than scrawny athletes, but children should not start trying to bulk up before they are the right age. The following pointers may help you understand or identify athletes who may be at risk for eating disorders:

- The better you know your athletes, the more you can help them. Watch your athletes for any physical, or possibly emotional, changes.

- Discuss nutrition issues, eating habits, and weight concerns openly. Encourage athletes to come to you with questions or to ask for advice.

> **Food should never be used as a punishment or reward.**

- If you think any of your athletes has an eating disorder or a distorted body image (believing they are fatter than they really are), let them know that they can come to you privately. Tell them that they can trust you to keep what they say confidential. They often want help but do not know whom to ask.

- If you identify a problem or feel unable to help, encourage the athlete to talk to his or her physician. Early identification and treatment are key to helping any athlete with an eating disorder.

The following pointers may help you prevent eating disorders:

- Adults should be role models for healthy attitudes toward eating and body image.

- Encourage children to eat according to their appetites. Never withhold food or force children to eat.

- Teach children to feel good about themselves, regardless of body size or shape.

Summary

Young athletes who receive nutrition and fitness education are less likely to develop eating disorders or body weight problems. Once they recognize that a certain percentage of body fat is healthy and even required for optimal performance, child athletes are better able to resist the temptation of becoming thin at all costs. Children can achieve a "competitive" weight through a sound, balanced diet and an appropriate training program. Whether trying to lose or gain weight, children need support and guidance from their parents, coaches, and health-care professionals.

CARBOHYDRATES: THE ENERGY BOOSTER

Q: Is there one BEST food for my child to eat in order to boost performance?

A: Instead of only one food, there is one best TYPE of food: CARBOHYDRATES. These foods are best because they are the preferred fuel for exercise. By feeding your child fruits and vegetables, low-fat milk and other dairy foods, and breads and cereals, you can be sure your child's diet contains adequate carbohydrates for performance.

Q: My child's favorite carbohydrate foods are ice cream and candy. Does it matter whether the carbohydrates are "simple" or "complex"?

A: Simple carbohydrates or simple sugars often taste sweet. They are easily digested and absorbed into the bloodstream to provide quick energy. Examples are milk, fruits, and "sweets" like candy and cookies.

Complex carbohydrates are starchy foods. They provide energy more slowly because they take longer to be digested. They carry other nutrients like fiber, vitamins, and minerals along with them. Because they carry these other nutrients, they are more healthful and should be eaten most of the time.

Q: I've always heard that carbohydrate foods like bread and potatoes are fattening. What is the real story?

A: Bread and potatoes are both excellent sources of carbohydrate. "Fattening" would only apply to these carbohydrates when eaten in excess quantity or with high-fat toppings such as margarine, sour cream, or bacon. If the excess energy was not required for the child's growth and activity, it would be stored as fat in the child's body.

■ ■ ■ ■ ■ ■ ■ ■ ■

Sample Menu Loaded with Carbohydrates

Meal	*Menu*
Breakfast	2 pancakes with syrup 1 c. low-fat (1%) milk 6 oz. orange juice
Snack	1 bagel with jam or jelly
Lunch	1 slice pizza Carrot and celery sticks 2 graham crackers 1 c. low-fat (1%) milk
Snack (Before practice)	2 fig bars

Sample menu continued

Snack (After practice)

1 box fruit juice
1 small box raisins

Dinner

4 oz. barbecued chicken
1 c. green beans
1/2 c. rice
1 piece French bread
Salad with 1 Tbsp. dressing
1 c. low-fat (1%) milk

Snack

1 c. low-fat frozen yogurt

■ ■ ■ ■ ■ ■ ■ ■ ■

PROTEIN: THE BODY'S BUILDING BLOCK

Q: How do the protein building blocks work together?

A: Protein building blocks come from the foods we eat. They work together to build and maintain the body. In other words . . .

Protein

- maintains and repairs muscle.
- makes hemoglobin which gets oxygen to the body.
- forms antibodies in the blood that fight off infection and disease.
- produces enzymes and hormones that regulate body processes.
- can supply energy when necessary.

Q: But I thought protein causes muscle growth, too. If protein doesn't, what does?

A: Protein does provide the building blocks for muscular growth, but muscular growth comes from a balanced diet, physical maturity, and training.

■ ■ ■

Basic diet

+

Level of maturation*

+

Training

=

Muscular growth

Q: How do I make sure my child gets enough dietary protein?

A: The Food Guide Pyramid suggests that children between the ages of 6 to 12 years get three (8-ounce) servings of milk daily and two to three daily servings of other protein foods such as meat, eggs, dry beans, and nuts. If the child athlete regularly consumes this, along with six servings of bread, rice, cereal, or pasta, and three servings of vegetables, his or her protein needs will be met.

* *Levels of maturation:* This depends on whether the athlete has reached the stage of maturation in which the hormones are released in sufficient amounts to add muscle mass.

High-Protein After School Munchies

■ ■ ■ ■ ■ ■ ■ ■ ■ ■ ■ ■

Crunchy Peanut Butter Sandwich

2 slices hearty, whole-grain bread
2 tablespoons crunchy peanut butter
2 tablespoons low-fat granola
1/2 banana, sliced

1. Spread peanut butter on the bread.
2. Sprinkle the granola on top of the peanut butter.
3. You may add sliced banana to soothe the sweet tooth.

Nutrition Information:
Calories 473, protein 17.2 g, carbohydrate 62.8 g, fat 20.8 g

Fruity Fizz

1 cup low-fat vanilla yogurt
1/2 cup berries (strawberries, blueberries, etc.)
1/2 cup seltzer

1. Combine yogurt and fruit in blender; blend well.
2. Add seltzer; blend again 2-3 seconds to fizz.

Nutrition Information:
Calories 227, protein 11.9 g, carbohydrate 39.3 g, fat 3.3 g

ATTACK THE FAT

Q: What is FAT?

A: Fat is a source of stored energy found in the muscles and under the skin. Fat is also found in many of the foods we eat—animal and plant foods. Each gram of dietary fat yields 9 calories. The majority of an athlete's dietary fat should be of the heart-healthy varieties; monounsaturated and polyunsaturated fats.

Q: Is it true that kids need a certain amount of fat to grow?

A: Yes. Kids do need dietary fat to grow appropriately. Fats are a source of essential fatty acids necessary for growth. Dietary fats also aid in the absorption of the fat-soluble vitamins A, D, E, and K. The American Academy of Pediatrics recommends that growing kids get an average of 30 percent of their daily calories from dietary fats.

Q: Can I trust food labels to give me guidance on low-fat foods?

A: In the past, many food labels did not tell the whole story. With the new food labels of May 1994, much of the confusion has been removed. Food labels can help you make healthy food choices for your family. Children often make high-fat food choices with convenience foods, but by reading food labels and becoming aware of serving sizes and fat content you can balance your child's plate. An occasional high-fat but nutritious food such as pizza can be balanced with a low-fat salad to help your child have a healthful diet.

■ ■ ■ ■ ■ ■ ■ ■ ■

FIGHT FAT ... THINK AGAIN

Breakfast

Instead of . . .	*Try . . .*
Sausage biscuit	Waffle with fruit
Hash browns	Grits or oatmeal
Whole milk	Orange juice
	Low-fat milk

Lunch/Dinner

Instead of . . .	*Try . . .*
Fried chicken sandwich	Grilled chicken sandwich without mayo
French fries	Pretzels
Chocolate cake	Apple
Regular milk shake	Low-fat yogurt shake

■ ■ ■ ■ ■ ■ ■ ■ ■

VITAMINS AND MINERALS

Q: Vitamins and minerals; are they magic or metabolic?

A: Vitamins and minerals are complex organic substances found in tiny quantities in the foods we eat. They do not contain energy but they do work together in the body to help maintain health and promote growth and development of children. So, they are not magic, but yes, they are metabolic and help the body function properly.

Q: If a little is good, will more be better?

A: Other than deficiency diseases, vitamins and minerals have not been shown to prevent or cure any disease, including the common cold. Supplementation will not cause the child to mature faster or become stronger. Encouraging supplementation is also teaching the child athlete to rely on a supplement as "insurance" of an athletic success rather than attributing the success to training, hard work, and a balanced diet.

Q: My child won't eat vegetables. Should I give a supplement to replace these nutrients?

A: Vitamin and mineral supplements should NOT be used to replace food or make up for poor dietary habits. The following table shows the great variety of food choices that supply the vitamins and minerals your child athlete needs.

Food Choices for Vitamins and Minerals

Potassium, vitamin C, A (if deep yellow)

Apples, apricots, bananas, cherries, fruit juice, grapes, peaches, pears, pineapples, plums, prunes, raisins

Iron, magnesium, phosphorus, potassium, folate, vitamins A and C

Broccoli, carrots, green pepper, kale, pumpkin, spinach, sweet potatoes, winter squash

Iron, magnesium, phosphorus, potassium, folate

Black-eyed peas, corn, lima beans, green peas, potatoes

Magnesium, potassium, folate, vitamins C and K

Cabbage, cauliflower, celery, cucumbers, green beans, lettuce, onions, summer squash, tomatoes, vegetable juice, zucchini

Potassium, folate, vitamin C, A (if deep yellow)

Oranges, grapefruit, cantaloupe, watermelon, strawberries, blueberries, raspberries, tangerines

Copper, iron, magnesium, phosphorus, thiamin, riboflavin, niacin, vitamin E

Brown rice, oatmeal, corn tortillas, whole-grain breads, whole-grain cereals, whole-wheat pastas and crackers

Iron, phosphorus, potassium, zinc, niacin, riboflavin, thiamin, vitamins B6 and B12

Beef, chicken, pork, turkey, ham

Copper, magnesium, phosphorus, vitamins A and B12

Peanut butter, seeds, almonds, walnuts, peanuts, other nuts

Calcium, phosphorus, vitamins A and B12

American, cottage, cheddar, part-skim mozzarella, ricotta, Swiss, and other cheeses

Iron, thiamin, riboflavin, niacin

Bagels, cornbread, grits, crackers, pasta, noodles, pita bread, ready-to-eat cereals, white bread, rolls

Calcium, phosphorus, potassium, riboflavin, vitamins B12, A and (if fortified) D

Low-fat milk, low-fat flavored milk, skim milk, buttermilk, whole milk

Iron, magnesium, phosphorus, potassium, folate

Black beans, chick-peas, kidney beans, lentils, navy beans, peas, pinto beans, soy beans

FLUIDS

Q: What is the best fluid to keep my child athlete hydrated?

A: Plain cold water is the best and most economical source of fluid. Cold fluids are absorbed faster than warm ones, and drinking water is the easiest way to rehydrate the body. It is a good idea to provide your child with his or her own water bottle.

Q: What about sports drinks?

A: Water is the best fluid to hydrate the child for practices and events lasting up to 90 minutes. If your child participates in long or all-day events, sports drinks or diluted fruit juices may be beneficial for carbohydrate replacement. The rule of thumb is 6% to 8% carbohydrate fluids; this means half-strength fruit juice, half-strength lemonade, and most sports drinks. Children may drink more if given a flavored fluid instead of water.

Q: How much fluid does it take to keep my child hydrated during sports events?

A: The child should be weighed before and after the exercising period to know how much fluid he or she lost. Then follow these basic guidelines to be sure your child is drinking enough because thirst is NOT an adequate indicator of the need for fluids.

Before Exercise	*During Exercise*	*After Exercise*
Drink 10 to 14 oz. of cold water 1 to 2 hours before the activity.	Drink 3 to 4 oz. of cold water every 15 minutes.	Drink 2 cups (16 oz.) of cold water for every pound of weight loss
Drink 10 oz. of cold water 10-15 minutes before the activity.		

Thirst Quenching Lemonade—During Exercise
6% carbohydrate solution

4 scoops of powdered lemonade drink mix per gallon of water

Nutrition information per 8-ounce serving:
Calories 51, carbohydrate 13.4 g

Thirst Quenching Lemonade—After Exercise
12% carbohydrate solution

8 scoops of powdered lemonade drink mix per gallon of water

Nutrition information per 8-ounce serving:
Calories 102, carbohydrate 26.9 g

EAT TO COMPETE

Q: There's a lot of talk about pre-event eating. What are the best pre-event foods for my child athlete?

A: Pre-event eating serves two purposes:

1. To prevent the child from feeling hungry.
2. To help supply fuel to the muscles during training and competition.

Eat	*Avoid Large Amounts*
Complex carbohydrate	Fat
Water	Protein
Moderate portions	Fiber
	Last-minute sweets

Q: Does it matter when my child eats a pre-event meal?

A: Yes, it is best for your child to eat a meal 3-4 hours before competition time. Your child may not feel well exercising with a full stomach. Carbohydrate snacks may be eaten up to one hour before the event. Some foods digest and leave the stomach quicker than others:

Fat-	4 to 5 hours
Protein-	3 to 4 hours
Carbohydrate-	2 to 3 hours, *but remember, carbohydrate foods that are high in fiber may take longer.*

Q: My child seems to have no appetite after hard training. Is it important that she eats immediately after the sports event?

A: The body is most receptive to replacing muscle carbohydrate, called glycogen, during the first 2 hours after hard exercise. It may be easier for your child to drink the carbohydrate rather than eat it. If this is the case, fruit juice or lemonade may be the answer. Sports drinks would be another choice, but most contain less carbohydrate than juice, and at this point, more is better. It is a good plan for the child to eat a high-carbohydrate MEAL within 5 hours after the event. Here are two suggestions:

> 1 large baked potato with grated low-fat
>   cheese and plain low-fat yogurt
>
> carrot sticks
>
> 1 cup fruit salad
>
> 1 cup low-fat milk

> 2 cups spaghetti
>
> 2/3 cup meat sauce with mushrooms and
>   peppers
>
> 2 pieces French bread
>
> 1 cup sherbet
>
> 1 cup low-fat milk

GOOD FOOD FAST

Q: My family eats out two to three times each week. How can I make sure my child gets nutritious foods?

A: Good news; in the past few years, fast-food franchises and family-style restaurants have taken healthful eating more seriously and have added more low-fat, nutritious food to their menus. Here are some ideas to help you and your child make informed food choices.

GO FOR IT!

Dairy foods
low-fat milk
frozen yogurt
low-fat milk shakes

Starches
bagels, English muffins
pancakes, waffles
cereals
bread sticks
baked potatoes

Salad bar
salad
carrot, celery sticks
pasta bar
fresh fruit
soups, not cream-based
low-fat dressings

Meats/main dishes
chicken filet
grilled chicken sandwich
chili with beans
plain hamburgers
vegetable pizza
chicken/turkey/ham/roast beef
 sandwich or sub

Beverages
fruit, vegetable juices
lemonade
low-fat milk

Sauces
catsup
mustard
barbecue sauce

CAUTION

Dairy
2% milk
soft-serve ice cream
milk shakes

Starches
small order French fries
corn bread

Beverages
diet soda
2% milk

Salad bar
chicken, tuna salad
coleslaw
macaroni/potato salad
cream-based soups

Meats/main dishes
cheeseburgers
steak sandwiches
cheese pizza

STOP (THINK AGAIN!)

Dairy
whole milk
hard ice cream

Starches
biscuit, croissant
large order French fries
   curly, cheese or other fries
pastry, pie or brownie

Salad bar
croutons
bacon bits
more than 2 Tbsp. of dressing

Beverages
regular soda
whole milk

Meats/main dishes
fried chicken
fried chicken sandwich
fried fish/fried fish sandwich
fish or chicken nuggets
"super," "deluxe," or "supreme"
   sandwich or burger
sausage, pepperoni or extra
   cheese pizza
bacon burger
breakfast biscuits (egg with
   sausage or steak)
sausage, bacon

Sauces
mayonnaise
mayo-type sauces
alfredo sauce
hollandaise sauce
added butter or margarine

98

THE WEIGHT BALANCE

Q: How do I know if my child is overweight, underweight, or at just the right weight?

A: There is NO one specific weight that is perfect for your child. Physicians and registered dietitians assess the child's weight by using national standards based on age and sex. There is an acceptable weight range for each increment of height of the child.

Q: Everyone says my child will "grow into his weight." Is this true?

A: It is normal for children to add extra body fat in preparation for the "growth spurt." But, if you are concerned about your child's weight, ask a physician and a registered dietitian to determine your child's growth potential and make recommendations for a healthy weight.

Q: My child has irregular eating habits and loves junk food. Should he be on a diet?

A: The childhood years are not too early to learn a prudent, heart-healthy lifestyle. Encourage your child to eat foods low in fat and high in complex carbohydrates like whole-grain breads, fruits, vegetables, and low-fat dairy products; to eat foods high in dietary fiber; and to avoid excessive salt in the diet. Daily physical activity is another heart-healthy habit that will allow your child never to worry about the "D" word: diet. Parents need to be role models to teach kids that physical activity and healthful eating can be fun.

For the overweight athlete . . .

Fat-Free Banana Muffins

Mix:
3 large well-ripened mashed bananas
2 egg whites
1/3 cup nonfat milk

Combine:
1/3 cup sugar
1 tsp. salt
1 tsp. baking soda
1/2 tsp. baking powder
3/4 cup whole-wheat flour
3/4 cup plain white flour

For the underweight athlete ...

Old Fashioned Banana Muffins

Mix:
3 large well-ripened bananas
1 egg
2 Tbsp. canola oil
1/3 cup low-fat milk (2% fat)

Combine:
1/2 cup sugar
1 tsp. salt
1 tsp. baking soda
1/2 tsp. baking powder
3/4 cup whole-wheat flour
3/4 cup plain white flour

For both recipes: Stir wet and dry mixtures together until moistened and lumpy. Spray cups of muffin tins with vegetable spray. Fill each cup 2/3 full, and bake at 350° F for 25 minutes or until toothpick inserted into muffin comes out clean. Each recipe serves 12.

Nutrition information:
Fat-Free Banana Muffins
Calories 106, protein 2.9 g, carbohydrate 24 g, fat 0.4 g

Old Fashioned Banana Muffins
Calories 142, protein 2.9 g, carbohydrate 26.8 g, fat 3.2 g

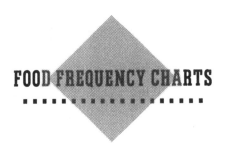

FOOD FREQUENCY CHARTS

If you plan to consult with a registered dietitian regarding your child's diet, it may be helpful to collect some information about what types of foods your child is eating. Use the food frequency chart to help your child determine how often he or she eats certain foods. Included on this chart are a wide variety of foods—some may be more healthful than others. The goal is to determine what foods are being eaten, so that a registered dietitian can interpret the chart and estimate nutritional adequacy. Just keep in mind that this is not necessarily a list of recommended foods.

Food	Usual portion size	Everyday (always)	3-4 times a week (often)	Once every 2-3 weeks (sometimes)	Don't eat (never)
Bread Group					
Biscuit					
Bread/roll					
Crackers					
Pasta/spaghetti					
Rice					
Potatoes					
Sweet potato					
Tortillas					
Bagels					

Food

Bread Group cont.	Usual portion size	Everyday (always)	3-4 times a week (often)	Once every 2-3 weeks (sometimes)	Don't eat (never)
Muffins					
Pancakes					
Waffles					
Cold cereal-presweetened					
Cold cereal-plain					
Hot cereal					
Pretzels					
Popcorn					
Other					

Food

Vegetable Group	Usual portion size	Everyday (always)	3-4 times a week (often)	Once every 2-3 weeks (sometimes)	Don't eat (never)
Carrots					
Corn					
Squash					
Green/lima beans					
Beets					
Peppers					
Broccoli/cauliflower					
Spinach/kale/collard greens					
Lettuce					

Food	Usual portion size	Everyday (always)	3-4 times a week (often)	Once every 2-3 weeks (sometimes)	Don't eat (never)
Vegetable Group cont.					
Tomatoes					
Tomato sauce					
Other					
Fruit Group					
Canned fruit					
Apple sauce					
Apples/pears					
Peaches/nectarines					
Oranges/grapefruit					

Food

Fruit Group cont.	Usual portion size	Everyday (always)	3-4 times a week (often)	Once every 2-3 weeks (sometimes)	Don't eat (never)
Melon					
Berries/kiwi fruit					
Grapes					
Bananas					
Fruit cocktail					
Fruit juice/drink					
Raisins/dates					
Papayas/mangos					
Other					

Food

Milk Group	Usual portion size	Everyday (always)	3-4 times a week (often)	Once every 2-3 weeks (sometimes)	Don't eat (never)
Cheese					
Skim milk					
Whole milk					
Cottage cheese					
Yogurt					
Frozen yogurt					
Ice cream					
Pudding					
Other					

Food

Meat Group	Usual portion size	Everyday (always)	3-4 times a week (often)	Once every 2-3 weeks (sometimes)	Don't eat (never)
Bacon/sausage					
Beef/hamburger					
Fried chicken					
Other chicken/turkey					
Dried beans/peas					
Eggs					
Fish/shellfish					
Liver					
Luncheon meats					

Food	Usual portion size	Everyday (always)	3-4 times a week (often)	Once every 2-3 weeks (sometimes)	Don't eat (never)
Meat Group cont.					
Nuts					
Peanut butter					
Pork/ham					
Hot dogs					
Other					
Combination Foods					
Pizza					
Tacos					
Casseroles					

Food

Combination Foods cont.	Usual portion size	Everyday (always)	3-4 times a week (often)	Once every 2-3 weeks (sometimes)	Don't eat (never)
Macaroni & cheese					
Frozen dinners					
Nachos					
Corn dogs					
Chili					
Fish sticks					
Soup					
Coleslaw					
Potato salad					

Food	Usual portion size	Everyday (always)	3–4 times a week (often)	Once every 2–3 weeks (sometimes)	Don't eat (never)
Combination Foods cont.					
Subs/hoagie sandwich					
Cheese steak					
Other					
Other					
Other					
Fats, Oils, & Sweets					
Cake/pie					
Candy					
Fig bars					

Food	Usual portion size	Everyday (always)	3-4 times a week (often)	Once every 2-3 weeks (sometimes)	Don't eat (never)
Fats, Oils, & Sweets cont.					
Cookies					
Butter/margarine/oil					
Low-fat mayonnaise					
Mayonnaise					
Low-fat salad dressing					
Salad dressing					
Pastry/doughnuts					
Potato chips/corn chips					
French fries					

Food	Usual portion size	Everyday (always)	3-4 times a week (often)	Once every 2-3 weeks (sometimes)	Don't eat (never)
Fats, Oils, & Sweets cont.					
Onion rings					
Soda (diet)					
Soda (regular)					
Syrup					
Sugar					
Honey					
Jelly					
Sweetened gelatin					
Other					

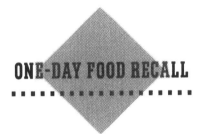

ONE-DAY FOOD RECALL

Everyone needs to eat food from the six food groups. It's especially important that young athletes consume a balanced diet. Ask your child to keep track of his or her food intake during the day. Or, work together with your child. Everything the child eats should be written down—putting just one food in each box. Review the appropriate sections in this book for food ideas. Use the example on pages 118 and 119 as a guide. With the help of a registered dietitian, the food recalls can be used to assess the balance and adequacy of your child's food choices.

BREAD group — 9 servings

1/2 Plain bagel	1/2 Plain bagel	Whole wheat bread (1 slice)	Whole wheat bread (1 slice)	Graham crackers	Pretzels
White rice	Popcorn	Oatmeal			

VEGETABLE group — 4 servings

Carrot sticks	Lettuce/tomato (on sandwich)	Coleslaw	Corn

FRUIT group — 3 servings

Orange juice	Raisins	Apple

MILK group 2-3 servings

2% Milk	2% Milk	Low-fat yogurt

MEAT group 2-3 servings

Turkey (sandwich)	Chicken breast	Peanut butter (on bagel)

Fats, Oils, & Sweets

Chocolate cookie	Mustard	Butter

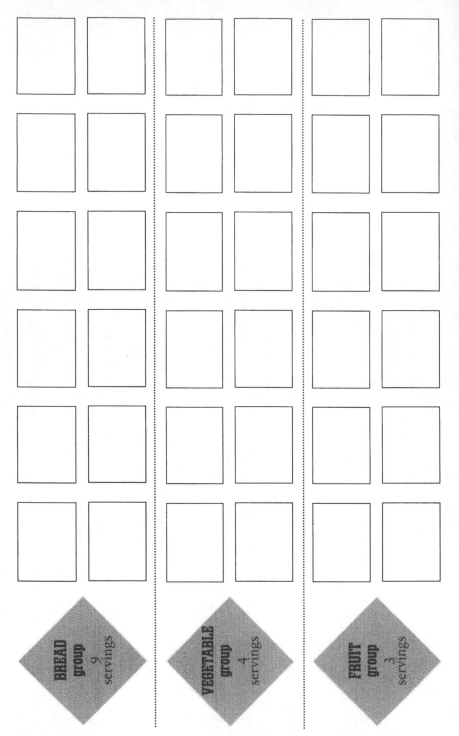

BREAD group 9 servings

VEGETABLE group 4 servings

FRUIT group 3 servings

MILK group
2-3
servings

MEAT group
2-3
servings

Fats, Oils,
&
Sweets

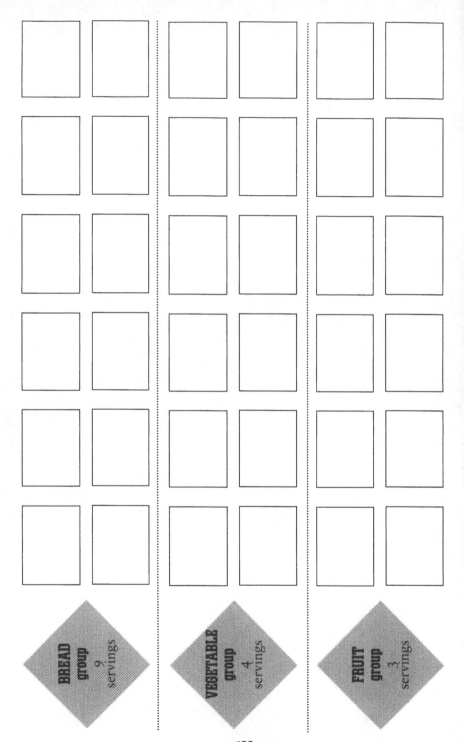

BREAD
group
9
servings

VEGETABLE
group
4
servings

FRUIT
group
3
servings

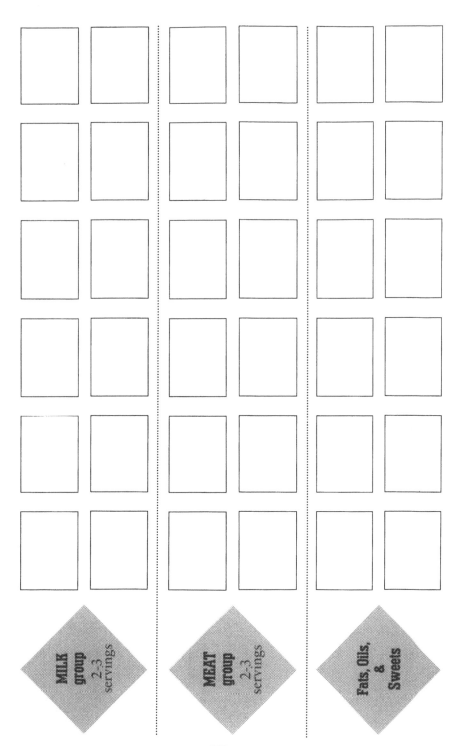

MILK group
2-3 servings

MEAT group
2-3 servings

Fats, Oils, & Sweets

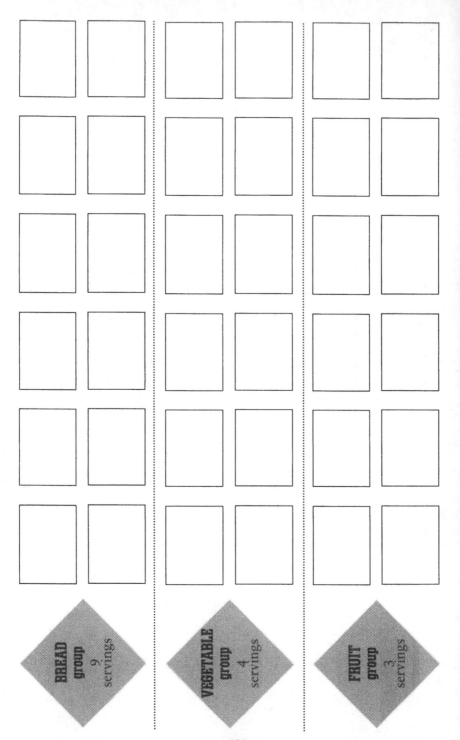

BREAD group 9 servings

VEGETABLE group 4 servings

FRUIT group 3 servings

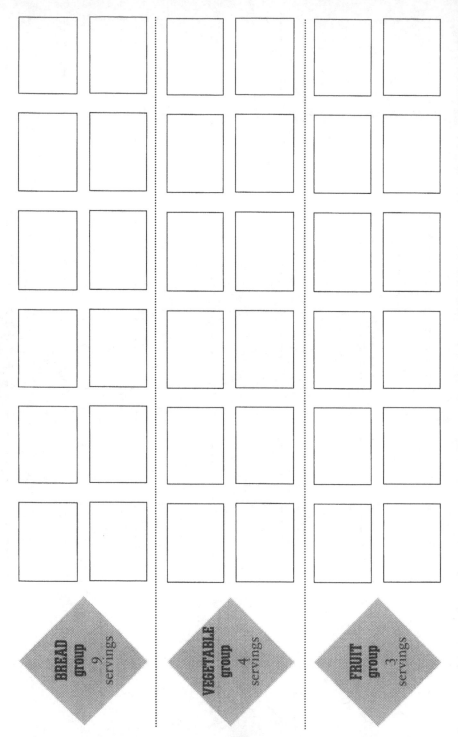

BREAD
group
9
servings

VEGETABLE
group
4
servings

FRUIT
group
3
servings

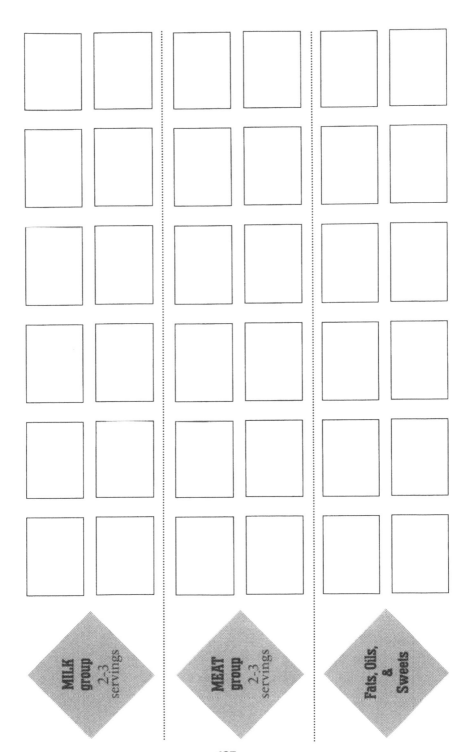

MILK group
2-3 servings

MEAT group
2-3 servings

Fats, Oils,
&
Sweets

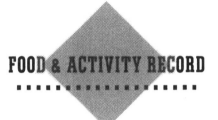

FOOD & ACTIVITY RECORD

Complete the following charts as accurately as possible, using the examples provided as a guide. Use only 1 form per day. Record everything the child consumes, including extras such as butter, mayonnaise, and jelly. Also, list his or her exercise activities and how he or she felt during the event (i.e., weak, energetic). Then, consult with a registered dietitian for an interpretation of the record and any recommendations for changes.

Date ———

Day 1—Sample Record

Time	Food	Type	Preparation	Amount	Activity	How did child feel
7am	Cereal	Corn flakes		2/3 cup		
	Milk	1%		4 oz		
	Bread	White	Toasted	1 slice		
	Jelly	Grape		1 tsp		
	Juice	Orange		6 oz		
11:15–12pm					Gym	Hungry
12:10pm	Pizza	Vegetable		1 slice		
	Carrot sticks	Fresh		1 carrot		
	Brownie			1 bar		
	Soda	Orange		12 ounces		
2pm	Granola bar	Plain		1 bar		
3:45pm	Apple			1 medium		

Day 1—Sample Record continued

Time	Food	Type	Preparation	Amount	Activity	How did child feel
3:45	Water			10 oz		
4-5pm					Soccer	Tired
5pm	Water			8 oz		
5:30pm	Chicken	Breast	Grilled	3 oz		
	Broccoli	Fresh	Steamed	1 stalk		
	Margarine	Tub		1 tsp		
	Rice	Brown		1/2 cup		
	Apple sauce			1/2 cup		
	Milk	Skim		1 cup		
8:30pm	Cookies	Chocolate chip		2		
	Milk	Skim		1 cup		

Date ———

Day 1

Time	Food	Type	Preparation	Amount	Activity	How did child feel

Day 1—continued

Time	Food	Type	Preparation	Amount	Activity	How did child feel

Day 2

Date ———

Time	Food	Type	Preparation	Amount	Activity	How did child feel

Day 2—continued

Time	Food	Type	Preparation	Amount	Activity	How did child feel

Date ———

Day 3

Time	Food	Type	Preparation	Amount	Activity	How did child feel

Day 3—continued

Time	Food	Type	Preparation	Amount	Activity	How did child feel

Day 4

Date ——————

Time	Food	Type	Preparation	Amount	Activity	How did child feel

Day 4—continued

Time	Food	Type	Preparation	Amount	Activity	How did child feel

Date ——

Day 5

Time	Food	Type	Preparation	Amount	Activity	How did child feel

Day 5—continued

Time	Food	Type	Preparation	Amount	Activity	How did child feel

Date —

Day 6

Time	Food	Type	Preparation	Amount	Activity	How did child feel

Day 6——continued

Time	Food	Type	Preparation	Amount	Activity	How did child feel

Day 7

Date ———

Time	Food	Type	Preparation	Amount	Activity	How did child feel

Day 7—continued

Time	Food	Type	Preparation	Amount	Activity	How did child feel

INDEX